ECG in 60 Minutes Emergency & ICU

High-Stakes Pattern Recognition for ER Nurses, Critical Care RNs & Rapid Response Teams

Ryan Mitchell, MD

Table of Contents

The 10-Minute Chest Pain ECG

A systematic bedside read under time pressure

ER NURSING · ACLS · RAPID RESPONSE

A patient arrives with chest pain. The ECG is in your hands. You have minutes — not the hour that a textbook chapter takes to read — to identify any life-threatening pattern, communicate it clearly, and initiate the correct action. This chapter is built for that moment. It does not add new content beyond what Books 1 through 4 have already taught. What it does is compress that content into a single, repeatable bedside workflow designed for real-time use under time pressure.

Everything in this chapter can be done in under 10 minutes. That is the target, and that is the standard the most effective emergency nurses in any department work to consistently.

1.1 The 60-Second Scan — Before the Full Read

Before applying the full 8-step reading method, every chest pain ECG deserves a 60-second triage pass that answers one question: is there anything here that requires me to act before I finish the systematic read? This is not a shortcut that replaces the full method — it is a safety net that catches the most time-critical findings while the full read is being completed.

THE BIG 5 — 60-SECOND TRIAGE PASS (from Book 3 Before Chapter 1, applied at the bedside):

1. Rate and rhythm: is there a wide-complex tachycardia, VF, bradycardia with hemodynamic compromise, or pulseless rhythm? If yes — act on the rhythm before continuing to Step 2.

2. ST elevation in ≥2 contiguous leads: is there ST elevation meeting threshold in any contiguous lead group? If yes — look immediately for reciprocal changes (Step 3) and confirm BBB status (Step 5) before calling a STEMI.

3. Reciprocal ST depression: is the ST elevation paired with mirror-image depression in the opposite lead group? Present = supports true regional STEMI. Absent = consider mimic (pericarditis, LVH strain).

4. Q waves — old vs new: pathologic Q waves with active ST elevation = current event. Pathologic Q waves without ST changes = old infarct; correlate with history.

5. BBB or paced rhythm: is the QRS wide? If LBBB or paced rhythm is present — stop and apply Sgarbossa criteria before reading any ST segment. Do not apply standard STEMI thresholds to a wide QRS.

WHAT THE 60-SECOND SCAN DOES NOT DO: It does not complete the diagnosis. It identifies whether the patient needs to be pulled out of the queue and acted on NOW, before the full systematic read is finished. Every patient still gets the full 8-step method — the scan just determines whether that method happens in 10 minutes or in 60 seconds.

1.2 The Full 8-Step Read — Applied at the Bedside

The 8-step reading method was introduced in Book 1 and applied in clinical detail in Book 3 Chapter 12. This section restates it in the compressed, action-oriented format appropriate for the ED setting — each step paired with the specific bedside decision it triggers.

Step	Check	Bedside Action if Abnormal
1	**Rate / rhythm**	Wide-complex tachycardia → prepare cardioversion. Pulseless → start ACLS. Bradycardia with compromise → atropine or TCP protocol (Chapter 2).
2	**Axis**	Unexpected left axis deviation in chest pain → LAFB? Old inferior MI? Extreme axis → lead reversal first (repeat ECG with correct lead placement before diagnosing pathology).
3	**Intervals**	PR > 0.20 s → document AV block degree. QRS > 0.12 s → STOP here, go to Step 5 (BBB check) before reading ST segments. QTc > 0.50 s → review all medications immediately.

4	**Chamber enlargement**	LVH voltage criteria met → the ST-T changes you are about to see in Steps 6-7 may be LV strain (not ischemia). Flag this before reading the ST segment.
5	**QRS morphology / BBB**	LBBB or paced rhythm present → SWITCH from standard STEMI criteria to Sgarbossa criteria. Do not apply standard thresholds. Calculate the modified ratio if concordant changes are absent (Book 3, Chapter 6).
6	**ST segment**	Apply correct threshold (standard OR Sgarbossa depending on Step 5). Check for elevation, depression, morphology (concave vs convex), and reciprocal changes. Nitrate pause: if inferior STEMI → V4R before NTG.
7	**T waves**	Hyperacute T waves → early STEMI, may precede ST elevation. Deep symmetric V2-V3 T inversion after resolved pain → Wellens (urgent cath, no stress test). Peaked tent-shaped T waves → hyperkalemia (check K^+ immediately).
8	**Clinical correlation**	Does the ECG match the story? Normal ECG in a convincing clinical presentation → serial ECGs and troponins, never discharge. Alarming ECG in a well-appearing patient → consider lead reversal, consider strain vs ischemia.

1.3 ST Elevation Triage — STEMI vs Mimic in Real Time

When ST elevation is found in Step 6, the next 60-90 seconds should answer one question: does this represent a true STEMI requiring cath lab activation, or a mimic requiring a different response? The following checklist is designed to be worked through in order, stopping at the first definitive answer.

ST ELEVATION TRIAGE CHECKLIST — WORK THROUGH IN ORDER:

1. Is the QRS wide (LBBB or paced)? If YES → standard criteria do not apply. Apply Sgarbossa. A positive Sgarbossa result = STEMI-equivalent; activate the cath lab.

2. Is the distribution REGIONAL (confined to a specific contiguous lead group)? If YES → move to Step 3. If the elevation is DIFFUSE (most or all leads) → go to Step 4 (pericarditis / Takotsubo / left main differential).

3. Are RECIPROCAL ST changes present in the mirror-image lead group? If YES → STEMI confirmed. Activate the cath lab. If NO but distribution is regional → proceed cautiously; still possible STEMI, but lower confidence without reciprocal changes.

4. Does the ST morphology suggest a mimic? Concave ('smiling') elevation + PR depression + NO reciprocal changes = pericarditis (NSAIDs + colchicine, not cath lab). J-point notching + concave + young asymptomatic patient = early repolarization (observation, not intervention).

5. Is the nitrate pause needed? Inferior ST elevation + RCA pattern (III > II, aVL ≥ I reciprocal depression) → obtain V4R before any nitroglycerin. V4R ≥ 1 mm = RV infarction = nitrates and diuretics are contraindicated.

THE MOST COMMON BEDSIDE ERROR IN STEMI TRIAGE: Activating a STEMI alert before checking for LBBB. A patient with known or new LBBB and chest pain has an ECG where standard STEMI criteria are unreliable — both false positives (unnecessary cath lab activation) and false negatives (missed MI) result from applying standard thresholds to an LBBB baseline. Always confirm QRS morphology in Step 5 BEFORE reading the ST segment in Step 6.

1.4 The Nitrate Pause — V4R and the 30-Second Rule

Nitroglycerin is one of the most reflexively administered medications in chest pain management. In the specific scenario of inferior STEMI with RV infarction, it is one of the most dangerous. The V4R check is the single nursing action that most consistently prevents this harm — and it takes approximately 30 seconds to obtain and read.

When to Obtain V4R

- Any inferior STEMI (ST elevation in II, III, aVF) — particularly when the RCA pattern is present (III > II, reciprocal depression aVL ≥ I).
- Any patient with inferior STEMI who is hypotensive or who becomes hypotensive after administration of a single sublingual nitroglycerin.
- Before the first nitroglycerin is administered in any inferior STEMI, as institutional protocol and best-practice standard.

How to Obtain V4R

- Place V4R at the right fifth intercostal space, midclavicular line — the mirror image of the standard V4 electrode, on the RIGHT side of the chest.
- Any of the standard limb leads (I, II, III, aVR, aVL, aVF) can serve as the V4R recording lead if a dedicated right-sided lead placement is performed. Most telemetry systems allow lead selection — use V1 position moved to V4R location.
- A positive V4R result is ST elevation ≥ 1 mm in the right-sided lead. This confirms RV infarction. The nitrate pause is now mandatory.

V4R Result	Action
V4R ≥ 1 mm (positive — RV infarction confirmed)	HOLD all nitroglycerin, morphine, and diuretics. Notify the physician immediately. Manage hypotension with IV fluid boluses (500 mL NS, repeat as needed). Vasopressors (norepinephrine) if fluids insufficient. Proceed with STEMI protocol (cath lab activation).
V4R < 1 mm (below diagnostic threshold)	Clinical caution still applies if the patient is hypotensive or the inferior STEMI appears large. Nitroglycerin may be given, but start at the lowest available dose, monitor BP continuously, and discontinue if BP drops ≥ 15 mmHg.

V4R not obtained before NTG given and BP dropped	This is the scenario the nitrate pause is designed to prevent. If it occurs: hold further NTG, place supine, 500 mL NS IV bolus immediately, obtain V4R now, notify physician urgently.

1.5 Communication — The STEMI Activation Call

Identifying the STEMI on the ECG is half the job. The other half is communicating it effectively to the physician, the charge nurse, and the catheterization laboratory in a way that minimizes delays and prevents errors. The SBAR format provides a reproducible, closed-loop communication structure for this call.

SBAR — STEMI ACTIVATION CALL

S — Situation: This is [Name], RN in the Emergency Department. I am calling about [Patient Name], a [age]-year-old [sex] in Room [X] who presented with crushing chest pain [X] minutes ago.

B — Background: Vital signs: HR [X], BP [X], SpO_2 [X]%. The 12-lead ECG obtained at [time] shows [X] mm of ST elevation in leads [X] with reciprocal ST depression in [X]. The pattern is consistent with [inferior/anterior/lateral] STEMI. [V4R was obtained and is negative/positive for RV infarction.] Troponin is pending. The patient is [stable/hemodynamically compromised].

A — Assessment: I believe this patient is having an acute MI and meets criteria for STEMI protocol activation.

R — Recommendation: I am requesting cath lab activation per our STEMI protocol and physician assessment at the bedside immediately. I am also notifying the charge nurse and preparing the patient for transfer.

CLOSED-LOOP COMMUNICATION: After delivering the SBAR, always confirm the physician has received the critical information: 'Can you confirm you are activating the cath lab protocol for this patient?' Wait for verbal confirmation. Document the time of the call, the physician who received it, and the verbal confirmation in the chart — this is both a patient safety and medicolegal requirement.

1.6 Telemetry vs 12-Lead — When Each Is Enough

A question that arises frequently in any busy ED or telemetry unit: when is a rhythm strip sufficient, and when must a full 12-lead be obtained? The answer is determined by what clinical question is being asked, not by the availability of the equipment.

Clinical Question	What Is Sufficient
Is this patient in VF, VT, or cardiac arrest?	Rhythm strip (telemetry lead II or any monitoring lead) — a 12-lead adds no additional information to the cardiac arrest decision and wastes time.
Is this tachycardia narrow or wide-complex?	Rhythm strip is sufficient for the initial narrow vs wide distinction. A 12-lead is then needed to apply the Brugada algorithm and classify the morphology.
Does this patient have ST elevation consistent with STEMI?	12-lead is mandatory — a rhythm strip covers only 1-3 leads and cannot assess the distribution, reciprocal changes, or territory required for STEMI diagnosis.
Is the bradycardia a sinus pause, Wenckebach, Mobitz II, or complete AV block?	A longer rhythm strip (ideally 60 seconds of a single lead such as lead II) is sufficient for AV block classification. A 12-lead adds axis and QRS morphology information that helps confirm the diagnosis.
Is this chest pain patient's ECG normal, improved, or worsened compared to the prior?	12-lead is mandatory for serial comparison — the same lead group must be assessed at each time point for dynamic change to be reliably identified.

1.7 Serial ECG Timing — When to Repeat and How to Compare

A single ECG is a snapshot. For any chest pain patient where the initial ECG is non-diagnostic, the serial ECG strategy is the most clinically important investigation the bedside nurse can drive — because the dynamic change between tracings, not the findings on any single tracing, is what most reliably identifies active ischemia.

Serial ECG Timing in Active Chest Pain

- Initial ECG: obtain within 10 minutes of triage registration for any chest pain presentation. Document the time of acquisition.
- During active symptoms: obtain a repeat ECG immediately when symptoms change (worsening, new quality, or localization change). Capture the ECG WHILE the patient is in pain whenever possible — this maximizes the chance of detecting dynamic changes.
- After symptom resolution: obtain a repeat ECG within 10-15 minutes of symptom resolution. Compare directly to the during-symptom tracing — changes that appear or resolve with symptoms are highly specific for ischemia.
- Fixed interval in non-diagnostic cases: in patients with ongoing but stable chest pain and a non-diagnostic initial ECG, repeat every 15-30 minutes for the first 2 hours.

What to Compare

- Always compare the current ECG side-by-side with the immediately prior tracing and the initial tracing on the same visit. The comparison to an initial tracing establishes the baseline; the comparison to the immediately prior tracing identifies dynamic change.
- Specifically look for: new ST elevation or depression, change in existing ST elevation or depression (≥0.5 mm change from prior is significant), new T wave inversion, new Q waves, or new conduction changes (new BBB, new AV block).
- Document WHAT changed, HOW MUCH it changed, WHEN the change was identified, and WHO was notified. The time-stamp of identification and notification is both clinically and legally important.

1.8 Documentation Standards — What the Chart Must Show

The ECG reading and the actions it triggers must be documented with a specificity that allows any provider picking up the chart hours later to understand exactly what was seen, when, what was done about it, and who was notified. The following documentation standard applies to any chest pain ECG that produces an actionable finding.

REQUIRED DOCUMENTATION ELEMENTS FOR EVERY CHEST PAIN ECG:

1. Time of ECG acquisition (not the time it was printed or read — the time the leads were applied to the patient).

2. Primary rhythm and rate: e.g., 'Sinus rhythm at 88 bpm.'

3. QRS morphology: 'Normal' / 'LBBB' / 'RBBB' / 'Paced.' This is documented first because it determines what criteria were applied to the ST segment.

4. ST segment findings: which leads, how many mm, morphology (concave/convex), and whether reciprocal changes are present or absent. E.g., '2 mm convex ST elevation in leads II, III, aVF with 1.5 mm reciprocal depression in I and aVL.'

5. V4R result (for all inferior STEMIs): 'V4R obtained at [time], [positive / negative] for RV infarction.'

6. Sgarbossa assessment (for all LBBB/paced rhythms in chest pain): 'Sgarbossa criteria applied. [Positive / Negative]. Modified ratio in V[X]: [value].'

7. Action taken and time: 'Provider [name] notified at [time] of ST elevation findings. Verbal STEMI protocol activation confirmed at [time].'

8. Comparison to prior ECG (if available): 'Compared to ECG on [date/time] — [new / unchanged / improved] ST changes.'

1.9 STEMI Activation — The Nursing Checklist

After a STEMI protocol is activated based on the ECG findings, the nursing role transitions from identification to preparation. The following checklist covers the standard nursing responsibilities before, during, and after cath lab activation — adapted to the specific needs of STEMI management in an ED setting.

Phase	Nursing Actions
Before cath lab arrival	Two large-bore IV accesses (antecubital, 18-gauge minimum). 12-lead ECG documented with acquisition time. V4R obtained and documented for inferior STEMI. Provider notification with SBAR documented. Aspirin 325 mg PO administered (confirm no aspirin allergy). P2Y12 inhibitor administered per institutional STEMI protocol. Heparin or anticoagulant per protocol. Chest X-ray obtained if time permits and does not delay transfer. Consent obtained (or documented as emergency circumstances).
Handoff to cath lab team	Verbal handoff with SBAR format: time of symptom onset, time of first ECG, ST findings, V4R result, medications given (drug, dose, route, time), allergies, vital sign trend, IV sites and patency, and any relevant history (prior PCI, known coronary anatomy, prior CABG).
Post-cath lab return (CCU transfer)	Vital signs on arrival. Continuous telemetry. Access site assessment (groin or radial). Post-ROSC care if arrest occurred (TTM status, MAP target, ventilator settings if intubated). 12-lead ECG within 30 minutes of return. First troponin post-intervention. Medication reconciliation (antiplatelet, anticoagulant, statin, beta-blocker).

BEDSIDE PEARL The bedside standard that experienced ER nurses reach first: by the time a physician is reading the ECG alongside you, you should already know the answer — and you should already have the V4R in hand if the inferior territory is involved. The 10-minute chest pain ECG is not about memorizing criteria. It is about running the same sequence every single time, without variation, so that when the difficult case arrives, the sequence runs on autopilot and the cognitive energy is available for the clinical judgment it requires.

KEY POINTS — CHAPTER 1

The 60-Second Scan and the 8-Step Method

- The Big 5 triage scan (rate/rhythm, ST elevation, reciprocal changes, Q waves, BBB status) identifies time-critical findings before the full systematic read. It does not replace the 8-step method — it precedes it.
- Step 5 (BBB check) must ALWAYS precede Step 6 (ST segment analysis). LBBB or paced rhythm requires Sgarbossa criteria — applying standard thresholds to a wide QRS produces both false positives and false negatives.

ST Elevation Triage

- Regional distribution + reciprocal changes = STEMI. Diffuse distribution + PR depression + no reciprocal changes = pericarditis. Concave + J-point notching + young asymptomatic patient = early repolarization.
- The nitrate pause: V4R before every nitroglycerin in inferior STEMI. V4R ≥ 1 mm = RV infarction = nitrates absolutely contraindicated. Replace with IV fluid boluses for hypotension.

Communication and Documentation

- SBAR format: Situation (patient, room, chief complaint) → Background (vitals, ECG findings) → Assessment (STEMI, needs protocol activation) → Recommendation (cath lab activation, bedside assessment now). Always confirm with closed-loop read-back.
- Documentation: time of ECG acquisition, QRS morphology first, ST findings with lead-by-lead detail, V4R result, Sgarbossa assessment if applicable, provider notification time, action taken.

Serial ECG and Telemetry

- Capture the ECG DURING symptoms when possible — dynamic changes during symptoms are the most specific finding for active ischemia. Compare every new tracing to the initial baseline and the immediately prior tracing.
- 12-lead is mandatory for STEMI assessment, serial comparison, and Brugada morphology classification. Rhythm

strip is sufficient for cardiac arrest rhythm identification and initial narrow vs wide distinction.

REMEMBER THIS

- ✓ Every chest pain ECG gets the same sequence every time: 60-second Big 5 scan → full 8-step method → ST triage checklist → V4R if inferior territory involved → SBAR call → documentation. The sequence does not vary based on how busy the department is or how certain the diagnosis appears. The cases where cutting steps seems most justified are the cases where the steps matter most.
- ✓ The nitrate pause is non-negotiable in inferior STEMI. A BP that collapses from 108/70 to 64/40 after a single sublingual nitroglycerin in an inferior STEMI patient is the most preventable hemodynamic complication in the ED. Thirty seconds to obtain V4R is always faster than treating RV infarction-induced hypotension after the fact.
- ✓ A normal initial ECG does not clear a chest pain patient. Up to 20% of confirmed MIs present with a normal initial tracing. The clinical story drives the workup — if the story is compelling, serial ECGs and troponins are required regardless of the initial ECG appearance. Document the normal findings, document the clinical reasoning for continued evaluation, and never use 'normal ECG' as a reason to discharge or deprioritize a patient with a convincing ischemic presentation.

Wide-Complex Tachycardia in the ED

VT vs SVT with aberrancy — the decision under pressure

ER NURSING · ACLS · RAPID RESPONSE

A wide-complex tachycardia on the monitor is one of the most time-pressured rhythm recognition scenarios in emergency nursing. The treatment pathways diverge dramatically based on a single assessment — stable or unstable — and the most consequential drug error in arrhythmia management (giving verapamil to a patient in VT) is also among the most common. This chapter gives you the bedside decision framework, the cardioversion technique, and the specific clinical traps that experienced ER nurses have learned to avoid.

The underlying ECG science (Brugada algorithm, AV dissociation, morphology criteria) is fully covered in Book 2 Chapter 5 and Book 4 Sections 4 and 9. This chapter applies those principles to the ED scenario: a patient on the monitor, a physician on the phone, and a decision that needs to happen in under two minutes.

2.1 The Stability Threshold — The First and Only Question

Before any attempt at rhythm classification, one question determines the entire management pathway: is this patient hemodynamically stable or unstable? This assessment takes approximately 15 seconds and overrides every subsequent diagnostic step. A hemodynamically unstable patient with a wide-complex tachycardia does not wait for a 12-lead, a Brugada algorithm calculation, or a physician-ordered medication — they get cardioverted.

Stability Assessment	Definition and Bedside Test

Hemodynamically UNSTABLE (cardiovert immediately)	ANY of the following present: (1) Systolic BP < 90 mmHg or signs of shock (pale, cold, clammy, altered perfusion). (2) Altered mental status not explained by prior baseline. (3) Ischemic chest pain (new pressure, heaviness, or radiation attributable to the rapid rate). (4) Acute pulmonary edema (new hypoxia, respiratory distress, crackles). One criterion present = unstable = cardiovert now.
Hemodynamically STABLE (systematic approach permitted)	All of the following: BP within acceptable range, alert and oriented, no ischemic chest pain, no pulmonary edema. A patient who is 'uncomfortable' or 'anxious' but meets all four criteria is still stable — proceed with the systematic approach (Section 2.2).

DO NOT LET A 'NORMAL' BP FALSELY REASSURE YOU: A BP of 102/68 in a patient who is pale, diaphoretic, confused, and barely responsive to commands represents hemodynamic instability — the numbers are a lagging indicator. The clinical picture overrides the cuff reading. If the patient looks unstable, treat as unstable.

2.2 The Stable Wide-Complex Tachycardia — Systematic Approach

In a hemodynamically stable patient, the systematic approach applies the Brugada algorithm to distinguish VT from SVT with aberrancy. The algorithm is applied to the 12-lead ECG obtained during the tachycardia — never to a rhythm strip alone, because correct Brugada application requires assessment of all precordial leads.

BRUGADA ALGORITHM — APPLY IN ORDER, STOP AT FIRST YES:

1. Is there ABSENCE of an RS complex in ALL precordial leads (V1-V6)? If YES → DIAGNOSIS: VT. STOP. (All precordial complexes are either purely positive or purely negative — no RS pattern in any lead.)

2. Is the RS interval > 100 ms in ANY precordial lead? Measure from the start of the R wave to the nadir of the S wave in the same lead. If YES → DIAGNOSIS: VT. STOP.
3. Is there AV DISSOCIATION? P waves marching independently at a rate different from the QRS rate, with NO consistent PR relationship. If YES → DIAGNOSIS: VT. STOP. (AV dissociation is pathognomonic of VT when present — no supraventricular rhythm can produce true AV dissociation.)
4. Do the QRS morphology criteria for VT apply? In RBBB-pattern: R monophasic in V1, QR or RS in V6. In LBBB-pattern: initial R wave > 30 ms in V1, notched S in V1-V2, Q or QS in V6. If YES → DIAGNOSIS: VT. STOP.
5. If ALL four steps are NO → DIAGNOSIS: SVT with aberrancy. Note: a Brugada-negative result makes SVT more likely but does not absolutely confirm it. Treat with caution (see Section 2.3).

AV DISSOCIATION IN PRACTICE: Looking for AV dissociation on a rhythm strip requires a longer strip than the default 6-second printout. Request a 10-15 second rhythm strip in lead II or V1. P waves marching through the QRS complexes at a rate independent of the QRS rate are the target — they appear as small deflections that walk through the QRS and T waves at regular intervals, occasionally producing a fusion beat (a hybrid QRS that looks intermediate between sinus and ventricular morphology) or a capture beat (a normally narrow QRS that briefly 'captures' ventricular conduction from the P wave).

2.3 The Wrong Drug Error — Why Verapamil Kills in VT

The single most dangerous drug error in the management of wide-complex tachycardia is administering verapamil or diltiazem to a patient who is in VT rather than SVT with aberrancy. Understanding the mechanism — not just the rule — is what produces the clinical instinct that prevents this error in borderline cases.

Drug	Effect in VT (Why It Kills)

Verapamil (IV)	Blocks cardiac calcium channels: (1) Vasodilation → drops systemic vascular resistance → precipitates hypotension in a patient whose BP is already being maintained by catecholamine compensation. (2) Negative inotropy → reduces an already-compromised ventricular function further. (3) AV nodal blockade → in a VT patient, this has no therapeutic effect (the VT is below the AV node). Net result: hemodynamic collapse and VF in minutes.
Diltiazem (IV)	Same calcium channel blocking mechanism as verapamil. Equally dangerous in VT. The common clinical error: a physician or nurse labels the rhythm 'narrow-looking SVT' based on a quick glance and orders diltiazem before a formal 12-lead is obtained. Never administer IV calcium channel blockers to a wide-complex tachycardia before VT is excluded with confidence.
Adenosine (diagnostic use in stable Brugada-negative)	Adenosine is not first-line for wide-complex tachycardia. However, in a hemodynamically STABLE patient where Brugada criteria are NEGATIVE and SVT with aberrancy is genuinely suspected, adenosine given as a diagnostic and therapeutic agent is acceptable — it will terminate SVT and has no sustained effect on VT. This is not a routine approach; it requires physician judgment and a Brugada-negative ECG.

THE RULE THAT PREVENTS THE ERROR: Treat every wide-complex tachycardia as VT until SVT with aberrancy is confirmed by a specific, identifiable mechanism — not because the patient 'looks stable' or 'the QRS doesn't look that wide.' Hemodynamic stability does not rule out VT. A normal BP in a wide-complex tachycardia is never sufficient reason to give verapamil or diltiazem.

2.4 Stable VT — Pharmacological Management

When a stable wide-complex tachycardia is identified as VT (or cannot be confidently excluded as VT), the pharmacological first-line agent is IV amiodarone. The cardioverter should be immediately available and the pads should be applied during drug administration — stable VT can become unstable VT within minutes.

Agent	Dose	Notes
IV Amiodarone (first-line)	150 mg IV over 10 minutes, then 1 mg/min × 6 hours, then 0.5 mg/min × 18 hours	Monitor BP during loading — amiodarone can cause hypotension from vasodilation. If BP drops significantly during infusion: slow the rate, give a fluid bolus, and cardiovert if the patient becomes unstable.
IV Procainamide (alternative)	20-50 mg/min up to 17 mg/kg total	Not first-line in structural heart disease or heart failure. Monitor QRS width during infusion — stop if QRS widens > 50% from baseline. More effective than amiodarone for some VT morphologies.
IV Lidocaine (adjunct)	1-1.5 mg/kg IV bolus, then 1-4 mg/min infusion	Less effective than amiodarone as first-line but widely available and fast-acting. Can be added if amiodarone alone is insufficient for recurrent VT.

2.5 Synchronized Cardioversion — Technique Step by Step

Synchronized cardioversion is indicated for any wide-complex tachycardia with a pulse in a hemodynamically unstable patient, and for stable VT that fails pharmacological management. The technique has several steps where errors frequently occur — the SYNC button, the energy selection, and the re-pressing of SYNC between shocks are the three highest-risk points.

SYNCHRONIZED CARDIOVERSION — STEP-BY-STEP BEDSIDE PROTOCOL:

1. Confirm the patient has a PULSE. If no pulse: this is DEFIBRILLATION (unsynchronized), not cardioversion. Do not use SYNC for pulseless patients.

2. Attach defibrillator pads: anteroapical position (right upper chest below clavicle / left lateral chest at the apex). Confirm good skin contact and pad adhesion.

3. Press SYNC ON. Confirm that the device is showing sync markers (small markers or arrows) appearing on the QRS peaks on the rhythm display — not on the T waves. If markers appear on T waves: adjust lead selection or gain until markers align with QRS peaks.

4. Select energy: Monomorphic VT: 100 J biphasic. AF: 120-200 J biphasic. Atrial flutter / AVNRT: 50-100 J biphasic.

5. Sedate if time permits: IV midazolam 1-2 mg or IV ketamine 0.5-1 mg/kg. Do NOT delay cardioversion for sedation if the patient is deteriorating rapidly — sedate if possible, cardiovert if not.

6. Clear the patient and bed: announce 'I am going to shock, everyone clear' and visually confirm no contact.

7. Deliver the shock. Note: synchronized cardioversion may have a brief delay (0.5-1 second) after pressing the discharge button — hold the button until the shock is delivered.

8. RE-PRESS SYNC after every shock. Most defibrillators automatically deactivate SYNC after shock delivery and revert to unsynchronized mode. Confirm SYNC is re-enabled before delivering any subsequent shock.

9. Assess rhythm and hemodynamics immediately post-shock. Document energy delivered, number of shocks, rhythm before and after, and hemodynamic response.

THE SYNC BUTTON IS THE MOST COMMONLY MISSED STEP: The automatic deactivation of SYNC after each shock delivery is a safety feature designed to prevent accidental synchronized delivery during VF. However, it means that every subsequent shock in a cardioversion sequence requires a deliberate re-press of SYNC. Delivering an unsynchronized shock to a patient in organized VT risks landing energy on the T wave (R-on-T) and triggering VF. This is avoidable with a deliberate checklist approach to every shock.

2.6 Post-Cardioversion Monitoring

Successful cardioversion does not end the nursing assessment. The 30-60 minutes immediately following cardioversion carry several important monitoring priorities that are directly related to the original arrhythmia and the cardioversion procedure itself.

Monitoring Priority	What to Assess and Document
Rhythm recurrence	Watch for return of the wide-complex tachycardia. Recurrent VT within the first 30 minutes requires: (1) IV amiodarone infusion initiation if not already running, (2) repeat cardioversion if hemodynamically unstable, (3) urgent cardiology consultation for recurrent or refractory VT.
Post-cardioversion 12-lead ECG	Obtain within 5-10 minutes of successful cardioversion. Identifies: underlying STEMI that may have triggered the VT (requires cath lab activation), baseline conduction abnormalities (LBBB, AV block), and QTc for arrhythmia risk assessment.
ST changes	New ST elevation or depression on the post-cardioversion ECG may reflect: demand ischemia from the tachycardia, a culprit STEMI that caused the VT, or post-cardioversion myocardial stunning. Any new ST change requires provider notification and troponin.
Hemodynamic recovery	BP, HR, and mental status should improve progressively after conversion. A patient who does not improve hemodynamically within 5-10 minutes of converting to sinus rhythm may have: a concurrent STEMI, severely reduced LVEF, or post-cardioversion myocardial stunning. Reassess and escalate as needed.
Transient post-conversion bradycardia	Expected and benign in most cases — the SA node requires a brief recovery period (overdrive suppression) after rapid tachycardia. If bradycardia persists (HR < 40 bpm) or the patient is symptomatic: atropine 0.5 mg IV.

Pad site assessment	Check skin under cardioversion pads for burns or erythema. Document pad placement, any skin changes, and patient comfort. Apply moisturizer or protective dressing if irritation is present.

2.7 Adenosine in Wide-Complex Tachycardia — When It Is Acceptable

Adenosine has a narrow, carefully defined role in wide-complex tachycardia. Understanding both when it is acceptable and when it is dangerous prevents the two most common errors: refusing adenosine in a genuinely Brugada-negative SVT patient (delaying appropriate treatment), and giving adenosine in an unconfirmed wide-complex tachycardia where VT has not been excluded.

Scenario	Adenosine Decision
Wide-complex, Brugada-NEGATIVE, hemodynamically stable, SVT with aberrancy genuinely suspected	Adenosine is acceptable as a combined diagnostic and therapeutic agent. If it terminates: SVT with aberrancy confirmed. If it does not terminate: treat as VT (amiodarone). Always have the cardioverter immediately available during administration.
Wide-complex, Brugada-POSITIVE or not yet evaluated, any hemodynamic status	Do NOT give adenosine until VT is excluded by Brugada criteria. VT may not respond to adenosine, and the transient hemodynamic effects (brief hypotension, flushing) can cloud the post-adenosine assessment.
Known WPW patient with wide + irregular + very fast tachycardia (pre-excited AF)	Adenosine is ABSOLUTELY CONTRAINDICATED. It blocks the AV node completely, forces all impulses through the accessory pathway at 300+ bpm, and can trigger VF. This is the highest-risk adenosine error in emergency practice.
Narrow-complex regular tachycardia (AVNRT/AVRT) in a stable patient	Adenosine is FIRST-LINE. This is the intended indication. Proximal IV site, rapid push, 20 mL saline flush immediately after.

ADENOSINE ADMINISTRATION TECHNIQUE:

1. Select the most proximal IV site available (antecubital fossa or more central). Distal sites (hand, wrist, foot) allow too much adenosine degradation before it reaches the heart.

2. Draw up adenosine 6 mg in one syringe and 20 mL normal saline flush in a second syringe. Set up both syringes at the IV port simultaneously.

3. Warn the patient: 'You will feel an intense chest tightness and flushing for about 10 seconds. This is expected and will pass.' Failure to warn produces extreme patient anxiety and makes the post-adenosine assessment harder.

4. Push adenosine as FAST as possible (1-2 seconds), immediately followed by the saline flush at maximum speed. The entire sequence should take < 5 seconds total. Slow administration allows adenosine to degrade in the peripheral blood before reaching the AV node in therapeutic concentration.

5. Record the rhythm continuously during and after administration. The characteristic post-adenosine sequence in SVT: brief AV block (flat line or severe bradycardia for 5-10 seconds) → sinus rhythm. In VT: no termination; the rhythm continues through the adenosine effect.

6. Be prepared for the brief post-adenosine period of AV block and possible short asystole (2-5 seconds) — this is expected and does not require intervention unless it lasts > 10 seconds.

2.8 Pre-Excited AF — The Wide Irregular Tachycardia Trap

Pre-excited AF in a patient with WPW is the wide-complex tachycardia that kills when mismanaged. It is wide, irregular, and very fast (> 200 bpm), and it superficially resembles AF with aberrant conduction or rapid VT. The difference is that the AV-node-blocking drugs appropriate for AF (adenosine, verapamil, diltiazem, digoxin) are immediately life-threatening in pre-excited AF.

PRE-EXCITED AF RECOGNITION AND EMERGENCY PROTOCOL:

1. Recognition: WIDE + IRREGULARLY IRREGULAR + VERY FAST (> 200 bpm) + known or newly suspected WPW. QRS morphology varies beat to beat (some beats more delta-wave-like, others wider). This combination is pre-excited AF until proven otherwise.

2. Hemodynamically UNSTABLE (BP dropping, confused, losing consciousness): IMMEDIATE UNSYNCHRONIZED DEFIBRILLATION 200 J. Do not waste time looking for SYNC markers in a rapidly changing polymorphic-appearing rhythm at 250 bpm.

3. Hemodynamically STABLE: IV procainamide 20-50 mg/min up to 17 mg/kg. Procainamide slows accessory pathway conduction without blocking the AV node. Defibrillator pads applied, defibrillator on standby at the bedside during infusion.

4. ABSOLUTELY CONTRAINDICATED: adenosine (blocks AV node → all impulses through AP at 300+ bpm → VF), verapamil (same mechanism + shortens AP refractory period), diltiazem (same as verapamil), digoxin (blocks AV node + shortens AP refractory period), IV beta-blockers (AV node blockade).

5. After termination: urgent electrophysiology consultation, ablation planning, and patient education on which drugs to avoid permanently.

2.9 Communication and Documentation

When a wide-complex tachycardia is identified, the communication to the physician must convey the key information needed for the cardioversion decision in a single clear statement. The documentation must capture the sequence of events with time-stamps that are accurate and specific.

SBAR — WIDE-COMPLEX TACHYCARDIA CALL

S: This is [Name], RN in the Emergency Department. Patient [Name], Room [X], [age]-year-old with a wide-complex tachycardia on the monitor.

B: HR [X] bpm, wide QRS [X] s, regular/irregular. BP [X], SpO_2 [X]%. Patient is [alert and stable / hemodynamically compromised — pale, BP dropping]. 12-lead obtained at [time] shows [QRS morphology, Brugada step result if completed, AV dissociation if present].

A: This appears to be [VT / wide-complex tachycardia of uncertain origin] and the patient is [hemodynamically stable / unstable].

R: I am requesting a physician at the bedside immediately. [If unstable: I am preparing for synchronized cardioversion now.] [If stable: Should I initiate IV amiodarone per protocol while you are en route?]

DOCUMENTATION MUST INCLUDE: Time of rhythm identification. Rate, QRS width, regularity. Stability assessment (BP, mental status). Brugada algorithm result (if applied). Cardioversion: time, energy, SYNC status, number of shocks, rhythm after each shock. Medications: drug, dose, route, time, response. Provider notification: name, time, verbal response. Post-conversion ECG: time obtained, findings.

BEDSIDE PEARL The most reliable clinical instinct in wide-complex tachycardia management: when in doubt, it is VT. Never give verapamil, diltiazem, or adenosine to an unconfirmed wide-complex tachycardia where VT has not been definitively excluded by Brugada criteria. The cost of treating SVT with aberrancy as VT (IV amiodarone when the diagnosis was SVT) is low — the patient gets a drug that is safe and may still convert the rhythm. The cost of treating VT as SVT (giving verapamil when the rhythm was VT) is hemodynamic collapse and potentially VF. The asymmetry of consequences makes the conservative default — treat as VT — the correct clinical instinct under pressure.

KEY POINTS — CHAPTER 2

The Stability Threshold

- ONE of: BP < 90 mmHg or shock signs, altered mental status, ischemic chest pain, acute pulmonary edema = UNSTABLE = synchronized cardioversion immediately. Do not attempt rhythm classification first.
- Hemodynamic stability does not rule out VT. A normal BP in a wide-complex tachycardia is never a reason to give verapamil.

The Brugada Algorithm

- Four sequential steps: (1) No RS in any precordial lead → VT. (2) RS interval > 100 ms in any precordial lead → VT. (3) AV dissociation → VT. (4) Morphology criteria → VT. Stop at first YES. All four NO = more likely SVT with aberrancy.
- Requires a 12-lead ECG, not a rhythm strip. Assess all precordial leads.

Drug Rules

- Stable VT: IV amiodarone 150 mg over 10 min, then infusion. Pads on, cardioverter ready during drug administration.
- NEVER give verapamil, diltiazem, or IV beta-blockers to an unconfirmed wide-complex tachycardia. VT + verapamil = hemodynamic collapse.
- Pre-excited AF (wide + irregular + > 200 bpm + WPW): procainamide IV (stable) or immediate unsynchronized defibrillation (unstable). Adenosine, verapamil, diltiazem, digoxin, and IV beta-blockers are ALL absolutely contraindicated.

Cardioversion Technique

- SYNC ON, confirm markers on QRS peaks (not T waves). Energy: VT with pulse 100 J biphasic. Sedate if time allows. RE-PRESS SYNC before every subsequent shock.
- Post-cardioversion: 12-lead ECG within 10 minutes, monitor for recurrence, amiodarone infusion for recurrent or prevented VT.

REMEMBER THIS

✓ Every wide-complex tachycardia is VT until SVT is confirmed by Brugada criteria. The 60-second stability assessment overrides all classification attempts: one sign of hemodynamic compromise = synchronized cardioversion now. Never let the search for a diagnosis delay cardioversion in an unstable patient.

✓ The SYNC button must be re-pressed before every shock in a cardioversion sequence. Most defibrillators auto-deactivate

SYNC after each shock delivery. A synchronized cardioverter that is not re-synced becomes an unsynchronized defibrillator, with risk of delivering energy on the T wave and triggering VF. Build the re-press into your sequence as a non-negotiable step.

✓ Pre-excited AF has an absolute contraindication list that must be memorized: adenosine, verapamil, diltiazem, digoxin, and IV beta-blockers. All block the AV node and force all fibrillatory impulses through the accessory pathway at rates exceeding 300 bpm, producing VF. The only pharmacological option for stable pre-excited AF is procainamide. For unstable pre-excited AF: immediate unsynchronized defibrillation.

Cardiac Arrest ECG Patterns

Shockable vs non-shockable — recognition to action

ER NURSING · ACLS · RAPID RESPONSE

Cardiac arrest rhythm recognition is the highest-stakes ECG skill in clinical practice. The interval between rhythm identification and the correct intervention is measured in seconds, and every additional second of delay in a shockable rhythm reduces survival by approximately 10%. This chapter is built around the two decisions that must happen faster than anything else in emergency nursing: is this rhythm shockable, and what happens in the first 10 seconds after the answer is known.

The underlying ACLS algorithms are fully presented in Book 2. This chapter focuses on the bedside application of those algorithms — the specific ECG features that allow rapid and accurate rhythm identification, the most common recognition errors, and the nursing role during each phase of the cardiac arrest sequence.

3.1 The Two-Category System — Shockable vs Non-Shockable

Every cardiac arrest rhythm falls into one of two categories that determines everything that follows. The category must be identified in under 10 seconds from the first rhythm check.

Category	Rhythms	First Action
SHOCKABLE (defibrillate)	Ventricular fibrillation (VF) Pulseless VT (any morphology)	Defibrillate 200 J immediately, then CPR 2 minutes. Time-to-shock is the most important determinant of survival in this category.

NON-SHOCKABLE (continue CPR)	Pulseless electrical activity (PEA) Asystole	Continue CPR immediately. Give epinephrine 1 mg IV/IO. Search for and treat reversible H's and T's. Defibrillating these rhythms wastes a CPR cycle and accomplishes nothing.

NEVER DEFIBRILLATE PEA OR ASYSTOLE: PEA is organized electrical activity without a pulse. Asystole is absent electrical activity. Neither has the disorganized re-entrant electrical circuit that defibrillation is designed to interrupt. Delivering a shock to PEA or asystole produces no benefit, wastes a CPR cycle, and can cause myocardial injury. If there is any doubt between asystole and fine VF, check lead selection, gain, and pad contact — then act on the most likely interpretation based on the best available signal.

3.2 VF — Recognition and Immediate Action

Ventricular fibrillation is the most common initial cardiac arrest rhythm in witnessed adult cardiac arrests and the rhythm with the highest survival potential when defibrillation is delivered within the first 1-2 minutes. Recognition is straightforward once the pattern is seen — but it must be distinguished from artifact, which is common in the chaotic environment of a cardiac arrest.

VF ECG Features

- Chaotic, disorganized waveform with no identifiable P waves, QRS complexes, or T waves.
- Amplitude varies continuously — waveforms are not uniform in height, width, or shape.
- Rate is effectively unmeasurable — the fibrillatory waveforms occur at 350-600 per minute but no organized rhythm can be identified.

- Coarse VF: larger amplitude fibrillatory waveforms (> 3 mm). Earlier in the arrest, more likely to be successfully defibrillated. Fine VF: lower amplitude (< 3 mm). Later in the arrest, lower success rate with defibrillation — ensure CPR quality is optimized to convert fine to coarse VF before the next defibrillation attempt.

VF vs Artifact

- Artifact mimicking VF: patient movement, lead disconnection, 60-Hz electrical interference. Key distinction: artifact typically has a regular, repetitive pattern (such as the regular sinusoidal waveform of 60-Hz interference), while VF is truly chaotic without any regularity.
- Check for a pulse while glancing at the monitor — if the patient is responsive or has a palpable pulse, any chaotic-appearing rhythm is artifact. If the patient is unresponsive with no pulse, treat as VF.
- Confirm with a second lead: artifact in one lead rarely appears identically in a perpendicular lead. True VF is global and appears in every lead simultaneously.

VF FIRST 2-MINUTE CYCLE — BEDSIDE SEQUENCE:

1. Identify VF (chaotic no-QRS pattern) and confirm no pulse: one check, under 10 seconds.

2. Announce 'VF — charging defibrillator' while CPR continues. Do NOT stop CPR to charge.

3. Charge to 200 J. Confirm pad contact and lead connection.

4. Announce 'everyone clear' — visual sweep of the patient, no one touching the bed or patient.

5. Deliver shock (UNSYNCHRONIZED — do not press SYNC for VF).

6. Resume CPR IMMEDIATELY after shock — do not check rhythm or pulse. Start 2-minute CPR cycle.

7. At the 2-minute rhythm check: if still VF — charge while CPR continues, shock, resume CPR. Give epinephrine 1 mg IV/IO after the second or third shock.

8. After the third shock: IV amiodarone 300 mg bolus. Second dose 150 mg if VF persists.

9. Continue 2-minute cycles: shock → CPR → rhythm check. Minimize hands-off time to < 10 seconds per check.

3.3 Pulseless VT — The Shockable Wide-Complex Arrest

Pulseless ventricular tachycardia has an organized, regular, wide-complex ECG appearance that can be visually mistaken for the pulse-present VT of Chapter 2. The only reliable way to distinguish pulseless VT from VT with a pulse is a pulse check — the ECG appearance alone is identical between the two.

VT Type	ECG / Clinical Features and Management
Monomorphic pulseless VT	Regular wide-complex tachycardia, uniform QRS morphology, no pulse. Management: defibrillate 200 J unsynchronized immediately (same as VF — do not use SYNC for a pulseless patient, as attempting synchronization wastes time and is unreliable in a rapidly deteriorating rhythm). CPR immediately post-shock. Amiodarone 300 mg after third shock.
Polymorphic pulseless VT (including torsades)	Irregular wide-complex tachycardia with varying QRS morphology and amplitude (twisting pattern in torsades). No pulse. Management: defibrillate 200 J unsynchronized. If torsades: also give IV magnesium sulfate 2 g after defibrillation, stop all QT-prolonging drugs, correct electrolytes. Note: do NOT use SYNC for polymorphic VT — the changing QRS morphology prevents reliable synchronization.

> **SYNC vs UNSYNC IN PULSELESS VT:** Synchronized cardioversion (SYNC ON) is for organized rhythms WITH a pulse. Pulseless VT has a pulse-verified absent status — treat identically to VF with unsynchronized defibrillation. Do not waste time pressing SYNC and waiting for sync markers to align on QRS complexes when the patient has no pulse.

3.4 PEA — Organized Rhythm, No Pulse

Pulseless electrical activity is both the most important non-shockable rhythm and the most frequently mismanaged one. Because PEA can show any organized ECG appearance — including a rhythm that looks like normal sinus rhythm — the error of defibrillating PEA or assuming a pulse exists because the rhythm looks 'functional' is common and dangerous. The pulse check is the only reliable PEA confirmation.

PEA Recognition

- PEA: organized electrical activity on the monitor, combined with confirmed absent pulse. The ECG alone cannot diagnose PEA — the rhythm may look like sinus rhythm, junctional rhythm, or any other organized pattern.
- Narrow complex PEA (QRS < 0.12 s): the organized rhythm is narrow, suggesting the conduction system is intact. The problem is mechanical — something is preventing the organized electrical activity from producing effective mechanical contraction.
- Wide complex PEA (QRS > 0.12 s): suggests more severe myocardial dysfunction or a metabolic/toxic cause. Associated with lower survival rates than narrow complex PEA.
- $ETCO_2$ monitoring during CPR: $ETCO_2$ < 10 mmHg with adequate CPR suggests very low cardiac output — typical of PEA from obstructive or distributive causes. A sudden rise in $ETCO_2$ to > 40 mmHg suggests ROSC even before a rhythm check is completed.

The H's and T's — Bedside Systematic Search

Category	Cause	Bedside Clue and Specific Treatment
H	**Hypovolemia**	Flat neck veins, trauma, blood loss → IV fluid bolus, blood products
H	**Hypoxia**	Cyanosis, low $ETCO_2$, inadequate ventilation → confirm BVM seal, advance airway, increase O_2

H	**Hydrogen ion (acidosis)**	Metabolic acidosis history (DKA, sepsis) → sodium bicarbonate 50 mEq IV, treat underlying cause
H	**Hypo/Hyperkalemia**	CKD history, ECG peaked T waves or wide QRS → calcium gluconate (hyperkalemia), dextrose + insulin (hyperkalemia)
H	**Hypothermia**	Cold body temperature, history of exposure → active rewarming, ECMO if severe
T	**Tension pneumothorax**	Absent breath sounds one side, deviated trachea, JVD → needle decompression 2nd ICS MCL immediately
T	**Tamponade**	JVD, muffled sounds, electrical alternans, low voltage → pericardiocentesis
T	**Toxins**	Drug ingestion history, pill bottles at scene → naloxone (opioids), sodium bicarbonate (TCA), Digibind (digoxin)
T	**Thrombosis (PE)**	Sudden arrest, recent immobilization, S1Q3T3, obstructive PEA (low $ETCO_2$ despite CPR) → tPA 50 mg IV bolus, continue CPR 60-90 min
T	**Thrombosis (MI)**	STEMI pattern on any available ECG → emergent PCI post-ROSC or during CPR if feasible

3.5 Asystole vs Fine VF — The Gain Check

Asystole is the complete absence of organized or disorganized cardiac electrical activity. It produces a flat baseline on the monitor. The danger is that the flat baseline of asystole can be mimicked by lead disconnection, very low monitor gain, or fine VF with very low amplitude waveforms. Treating fine VF as asystole (not defibrillating) is a potentially reversible error; treating asystole as fine VF (defibrillating a flat line) wastes a CPR cycle.

ASYSTOLE CONFIRMATION PROTOCOL — DO ALL THREE BEFORE CALLING ASYSTOLE:

1. Check gain: increase the monitor gain to maximum. Fine VF waveforms that appeared flat at standard gain may become visible at higher gain.

2. Check lead selection: switch to a different lead (e.g., from lead II to lead I or lead III). Fine VF typically persists across multiple leads; lead disconnection artifact usually disappears in a different lead.

3. Check pad/lead contact: confirm pads are firmly adherent to clean, dry skin. Verify lead cable connections. A disconnected pad produces a flat baseline on the affected channel.

4. If all three checks confirm a truly flat baseline with no detectable waveforms: this is asystole. Continue CPR, give epinephrine 1 mg IV/IO every 3-5 minutes, search for H's and T's. Do not defibrillate asystole.

WHY THIS MATTERS: Fine VF (low-amplitude fibrillatory waveforms < 3 mm) is a shockable rhythm that responds to defibrillation. Incorrectly classifying it as asystole and not defibrillating removes the patient's only path to rhythm restoration from the shockable pathway. The gain check adds 10 seconds to the rhythm check but may be the difference between a correct and incorrect treatment decision.

3.6 Post-ROSC ECG Triage

When return of spontaneous circulation (ROSC) is achieved, the ECG obtained immediately post-ROSC is one of the most actionable findings in the entire resuscitation. It identifies the underlying cause of the arrest, guides the decision for emergent catheterization, and directs the initial post-ROSC care priorities.

Post-ROSC ECG Finding	Action and Priority
ST elevation (any STEMI pattern)	Activate the cath lab for emergent PCI. Do NOT delay for neurological assessment — neurological prognosis cannot be reliably assessed acutely and should never delay PCI when ST elevation is present. Begin TTM (targeted temperature management) simultaneously if the patient is comatose (GCS < 8, not following commands).
LBBB (new or unknown age) + chest pain preceded arrest	Apply Sgarbossa criteria immediately (Book 3, Chapter 6). If Sgarbossa-positive: activate the cath lab (treat as STEMI-equivalent). If Sgarbossa-negative: serial ECGs and troponins; cardiology consultation for angiography decision.
Normal ECG	Does not exclude a coronary cause of arrest. Coronary angiography remains appropriate for most comatose post-VF arrest patients without a clear identified non-coronary cause. Serial troponins to identify rising injury markers.
Diffuse ST depression + aVR elevation	Left main or severe multivessel disease as the arrest trigger. Highest-risk post-ROSC coronary anatomy. Emergent angiography with circulatory support (IABP/Impella) preparation.
Complete AV block with wide ventricular escape	Transcutaneous pacing immediately (atropine will not work for wide escape). Cardiology consultation for transvenous pacing and permanent device evaluation.
Electrical alternans + low voltage	Tamponade may have caused or complicated the arrest. Bedside echocardiography urgently; pericardiocentesis if confirmed.

3.7 $ETCO_2$ as a Resuscitation Guide

End-tidal CO_2 ($ETCO_2$) monitoring during cardiac arrest provides real-time information about CPR quality and the likelihood of ROSC that the ECG alone cannot provide. In any intubated or supraglottic-airway patient, $ETCO_2$ monitoring should be continuous throughout the arrest.

$ETCO_2$ Finding	Clinical Interpretation
$ETCO_2$ < 10 mmHg despite adequate CPR	Very low cardiac output. Two possibilities: (1) CPR quality is inadequate (depth, rate, recoil) — reassess compressor technique. (2) The underlying cause is obstructive (PE, tamponade) — escalate H's and T's search urgently.
$ETCO_2$ 10-30 mmHg during CPR	Marginal but present cardiac output from CPR. Normal range during effective CPR — confirms adequate compression depth and rate.
Sudden rise in $ETCO_2$ to ≥ 40 mmHg	ROSC — the sudden dramatic rise reflects the heart resuming its role in CO_2 delivery to the lungs. Pause CPR immediately and check for pulse and rhythm. Do not wait for the scheduled 2-minute rhythm check when this occurs.
$ETCO_2$ consistently < 10 mmHg after 20+ minutes of optimal CPR	Associated with very low probability of ROSC. This finding, combined with the clinical context (unwitnessed, prolonged downtime, no reversible cause identified), informs the discussion of resuscitation termination — but does not by itself constitute a criteria for stopping.

3.8 Hypothermic Arrest — Modified ACLS

Cardiac arrest in the setting of severe hypothermia (core temperature < 30°C) requires specific modifications to standard ACLS, because the hypothermic myocardium behaves differently from the normothermic heart in every aspect of the resuscitation.

HYPOTHERMIC CARDIAC ARREST — MODIFIED ACLS PROTOCOL:

1. Continue CPR without interruption — the hypothermic myocardium can survive prolonged arrest with dramatically reduced metabolic demands. Do NOT terminate resuscitation based on time alone: 'not dead until warm and dead.'

2. Defibrillation: attempt defibrillation at standard energy (200 J). If temperature < 30°C and defibrillation fails after 3 attempts, defer further shocks until core temperature > 30°C (the myocardium is resistant to defibrillation below this threshold). Continue CPR and active rewarming between attempts.

3. Withhold epinephrine and amiodarone until core temperature > 30°C: at very low temperatures, drug metabolism is severely impaired — repeated doses accumulate to toxic levels and can produce drug toxicity upon rewarming. Resume at standard intervals once temperature exceeds 30°C.

4. Active rewarming: warm humidified oxygen, warm IV fluids (42°C), external warming blankets. Preferred for severe hypothermic arrest: ECMO (extracorporeal membrane oxygenation) rewarming — provides both CPR support and active core rewarming simultaneously. If ECMO is available, it should be considered for any patient in hypothermic cardiac arrest.

5. Target: restore core temperature to > 32°C before pronouncing death. Patients have survived neurologically intact after > 6 hours of hypothermic CPR — the rewarming goal is the exit criterion from resuscitation, not a time limit.

3.9 Nursing Role During Cardiac Arrest — Team Positions

Effective cardiac arrest management depends on role clarity as much as clinical knowledge. When every team member knows their position before the arrest begins, the resuscitation runs faster and more smoothly than when roles are assigned in real time. The following describes the standard nursing role assignments during a two-nurse cardiac arrest response.

Role	Responsibilities

Compressor (Nurse 1)	High-quality CPR: depth 5-6 cm (2-2.4 inches), rate 100-120 per minute, full chest recoil, minimize hands-off time. Switch compressors every 2 minutes (at rhythm check) to prevent fatigue-related quality decline. Announce fatigue immediately if it occurs before the 2-minute interval.
Defibrillator/ Medication Nurse (Nurse 2)	Apply pads. Operate the defibrillator (charge, clear, deliver). Draw and administer medications per protocol (epinephrine, amiodarone). Monitor rhythm display and announce rhythm at each check. Document all interventions with time-stamps. Communicate with the team leader (physician) on rhythm status and protocol progress.
Team Leader (Physician or senior RN)	Direct the resuscitation. Assign roles. Make decisions on H's and T's investigations. Determine rhythm at each check. Decide on specialty interventions (pericardiocentesis, intubation, ECMO referral). Communicate with family.
Airway Manager	BVM or advanced airway management. Confirm airway position with $ETCO_2$ and chest rise. Monitor ventilation rate (10 breaths/min with advanced airway). Call out any airway concern immediately.

BEDSIDE PEARL The number that most changes bedside behavior: every 1 minute of delay to defibrillation in witnessed VF reduces survival by approximately 10%. For an AED-accessible institution, a patient in VF at the nursing station should receive the first shock within 3 minutes. The only thing standing between that patient and the best possible outcome is the time it takes to confirm no pulse, call for the defibrillator, attach the pads, and charge. Practice the sequence until it runs in under 60 seconds. That is the standard.

KEY POINTS — CHAPTER 3

Shockable vs Non-Shockable

- Shockable (VF, pulseless VT): defibrillate 200 J immediately, then CPR 2 minutes. Time-to-shock is the primary determinant of survival. Do not delay for rhythm classification beyond the pulse check.

- Non-shockable (PEA, asystole): CPR + epinephrine 1 mg every 3-5 minutes + H's and T's search. Never defibrillate PEA or asystole.

Recognition Accuracy

- VF vs artifact: confirm in two perpendicular leads, correlate with pulse check. Artifact has regularity; VF is truly chaotic.
- Asystole vs fine VF: check gain, switch leads, verify pad contact before calling asystole. Missing fine VF removes the patient from the shockable pathway.
- PEA requires a pulse check — the ECG appearance alone cannot confirm or exclude PEA. Any organized rhythm without a pulse is PEA.

Post-ROSC ECG

- ST elevation → emergent PCI without waiting for neurological assessment. LBBB → Sgarbossa criteria. Normal ECG does not exclude coronary cause.
- $ETCO_2$ sudden rise to ≥ 40 mmHg during CPR = ROSC — pause CPR and check pulse immediately without waiting for the scheduled 2-minute check.

Hypothermic Arrest

- 'Not dead until warm and dead.' Continue CPR regardless of downtime. Withhold drugs below 30°C. Up to 3 defibrillation attempts acceptable; defer further shocks until temperature > 30°C. ECMO rewarming is the preferred method for severe cases.

REMEMBER THIS

✓ The two-category decision (shockable vs non-shockable) must happen in under 10 seconds from the first rhythm check. VF and pulseless VT get immediate defibrillation — nothing else happens first. PEA and asystole get CPR and H's and T's — defibrillation of these rhythms accomplishes nothing. The category, not the specific rhythm name, drives every subsequent action.

- ✓ $ETCO_2$ is the real-time window into CPR effectiveness and ROSC status that the ECG alone cannot provide. A sudden rise to ≥ 40 mmHg during CPR is ROSC until proven otherwise — pause CPR and check for a pulse immediately, even mid-cycle. A value persistently < 10 mmHg despite optimal technique suggests either an obstructive cause (PE, tamponade) requiring specific treatment or poor perfusion from severe underlying pathology.
- ✓ The post-ROSC 12-lead ECG is the next critical ECG decision point after the arrest rhythm. ST elevation on the post-ROSC ECG triggers emergent PCI without delay for neurological assessment — prognosis cannot be reliably assessed acutely. A normal post-ROSC ECG does not exclude a coronary cause and does not prevent angiography in a comatose post-VF arrest patient.

High-Risk Patterns the First Nurse Must Not Miss

Wellens, de Winter, left main, pre-excited AF, posterior MI, electrical alternans

ER NURSING · ACLS · NCLEX

Six ECG patterns are responsible for a disproportionate share of preventable cardiac deaths in the emergency department. What makes them dangerous is not that they are rare or complex — it is that they look, at first glance, like something benign. The patient whose ECG shows Wellens syndrome is often pain-free and appears well. The patient with de Winter pattern has no ST elevation. The patient in pre-excited AF may be alert and talking. In each case, the first nurse who reads the ECG is the last reliable safety check before a catastrophic outcome.

This chapter presents each pattern in a format designed for rapid bedside recognition: what it looks like at first glance, what the specific ECG clue actually is, the most common trap that leads to the wrong action, and the correct action. All six patterns require an action more urgent than 'observe and recheck in an hour.'

4.1 Wellens Syndrome

Wellens syndrome is one of the most dangerous ECG patterns in emergency medicine precisely because it appears when the patient is feeling better. The chest pain has resolved, the patient may look comfortable, and the ECG shows no ST elevation — yet the finding on that tracing indicates a critical, flow-limiting proximal LAD stenosis that will re-occlude and cause a massive anterior STEMI without urgent intervention.

WELLENS SYNDROME

LOOKS LIKE: A comfortable, pain-free patient whose chest pain has resolved. ECG appears reassuring — no ST elevation, no Q waves. Provider suggests stress testing for further risk stratification.

ECG CLUE: Deep, symmetric T wave inversion in V2-V3 (Type A — most common), or biphasic T waves in V2-V3 (Type B). These T wave changes appear in the pain-FREE state, not during active chest pain. They reflect reperfusion of the LAD territory after transient spontaneous occlusion.

THE TRAP: Ordering a stress test. The Wellens pattern identifies a critical proximal LAD stenosis that has temporarily reperfused — the stress test-induced ischemia can trigger a massive anterior STEMI during the test, in the radiology suite, away from the resuscitation team.

ACTION: Urgent cardiology consultation and NPO status. The patient requires coronary angiography on an urgent basis — not stress testing, not discharge with cardiology follow-up, not observation with serial troponins alone. Communicate the Wellens pattern directly to the physician by name. Document the communication.

Feature	Type A (Classic)	Type B
T wave morphology	Deep, symmetric T wave inversion — both upstroke and downstroke are equally steep; the nadir is at the center of the T wave	Biphasic T wave — initially positive (upright) then negative, with the terminal portion below baseline
Location	V2-V3 (occasionally extending to V4)	V2-V3 (same distribution as Type A)
Clinical timing	Present in the pain-FREE state after resolved chest pain	Present in the pain-FREE state after resolved chest pain
Significance	Critical proximal LAD stenosis — same urgency regardless of type	Critical proximal LAD stenosis — same urgency regardless of type

THE STRESS TEST TRAP: The Wellens pattern is an absolute contraindication to stress testing. The pathophysiology: the LAD stenosis is severe enough to produce spontaneous transient occlusion at rest. Exercise-induced catecholamine surges and increased myocardial demand during a stress test can trigger re-occlusion of the LAD, producing a massive anterior STEMI with the patient in the treadmill room rather than in the resuscitation bay. Communicate this directly to any provider who suggests stress testing for a Wellens patient.

4.2 De Winter Pattern

The de Winter pattern is the anterior STEMI that does not show ST elevation. It represents proximal LAD occlusion with a specific electrophysiological variant that bypasses the classic ST elevation stage, producing instead a pattern of upsloping ST depression combined with tall peaked T waves in the precordial leads. Because it lacks ST elevation, it will be missed by any STEMI alert system that relies solely on ST elevation criteria — and the first nurse to read the ECG is the primary safety net.

DE WINTER PATTERN

LOOKS LIKE: A patient with crushing anterior chest pain whose ECG is flagged as 'no ST elevation — possible NSTEMI.' Provider suggests serial troponins and admission.

ECG CLUE: In leads V1-V4: upsloping ST segment depression at the J point (1-3 mm below baseline, rising upward from the J point toward a tall, peaked, symmetric T wave). The T waves are strikingly tall and narrow-based. Often accompanied by 1-2 mm ST elevation in aVR. No ST elevation in V1-V6.

THE TRAP: Admitting as NSTEMI and waiting for troponin results. The de Winter pattern represents an acute LAD occlusion — it requires the same door-to-balloon urgency as any other anterior STEMI. The troponin will be elevated (or will rise), but waiting for it adds hours of ongoing myocardial necrosis.

ACTION: STEMI-equivalent protocol activation. Treat as a proximal LAD occlusion with the same urgency as V1-V4 ST elevation. Notify the physician immediately using the specific pattern name — 'de Winter pattern, requesting cath lab activation.' Document the time of identification and the communication.

HOW TO RECOGNIZE IT AT THE BEDSIDE: The key visual clue in de Winter pattern: the ST segment does not stay flat or go straight down from the J point as it does in ischemic ST depression — it RISES upward from the J point and continues rising into an unusually tall, peaked T wave. The J point is below baseline (depressed), but the T wave is above baseline and larger than expected. This upsloping ST-to-tall-T configuration in V1-V4, in the context of anterior chest pain, is the de Winter pattern.

4.3 Left Main / Diffuse Subendocardial Ischemia

The left main coronary artery pattern is the highest-risk STEMI equivalent in this chapter. It produces none of the dramatic regional ST elevation that standard STEMI criteria look for — instead, it shows widespread ST depression across most of the 12-lead, with a paradoxical ST elevation specifically in lead aVR. The combination reflects global subendocardial ischemia from critically reduced perfusion of the entire left ventricle.

LEFT MAIN / SEVERE MULTIVESSEL DISEASE PATTERN

LOOKS LIKE: A patient with chest pain and 'non-specific ST depression' across multiple leads. The ECG looks busy but not dramatic. Provider considers NSTEMI workup with serial troponins.

ECG CLUE: ST depression in ≥6-8 leads simultaneously (typically V2-V6, I, II, aVL), with ST elevation ONLY in lead aVR (≥1 mm) and sometimes also V1. No regional ST elevation in any standard STEMI territory. The distribution is the opposite of a focal STEMI — depression everywhere, elevation only in aVR.

THE TRAP: Treating this as routine NSTEMI with serial troponin evaluation. This pattern identifies left main or severe triple-vessel disease — the most hostile coronary anatomy possible. The absence of regional ST elevation does not reduce the urgency. These patients require the same door-to-catheterization urgency as a standard STEMI.

ACTION: **Urgent cardiology consultation for emergent or same-day coronary angiography. This is not a 'serial troponin and evaluate tomorrow' situation. Communicate the aVR elevation and diffuse depression pattern to the physician explicitly. Prepare for hemodynamic monitoring and possible circulatory support — these patients can deteriorate rapidly.**

Feature	Detail
aVR elevation mechanism	Lead aVR views the base of the heart from a unique vantage point. When global subendocardial ischemia generates a ST vector pointing toward the cardiac base (away from the widespread ischemic zone), aVR is the only lead that faces this vector directly, showing elevation while every other lead shows depression.
Minimum depression threshold	ST depression in ≥6 leads is the widely cited threshold for suspecting left main or multivessel disease. The more leads with depression, and the greater the magnitude of aVR elevation, the more strongly this anatomy is implicated.
Hemodynamic range	This pattern can appear in a patient with a systolic BP of 140 mmHg (compensated) or 60 mmHg (cardiogenic shock). Hemodynamic stability does not reduce the urgency of the anatomical implication.
Troponin timing	Troponin will be elevated or will rise, but waiting for it to confirm severity before escalating misunderstands the role of troponin in this context. The ECG pattern itself is sufficient to escalate.

4.4 Pre-Excited AF — Wide Irregular Very Fast Tachycardia in WPW

Pre-excited AF is covered in Chapter 2 in the context of wide-complex tachycardia management. It is included in this chapter as well because the specific nursing intervention that prevents the most catastrophic outcome — holding adenosine, verapamil, diltiazem, and digoxin — must be recognizable from the ECG pattern alone, before a physician is at the bedside and before any medication order is received.

PRE-EXCITED AF

LOOKS LIKE: A fast, irregular tachycardia in a patient with a prior WPW diagnosis (or on a prior ECG showing short PR and delta waves). The monitor shows what looks like rapid AF. A provider on the phone orders IV diltiazem for rate control.

ECG CLUE: WIDE + IRREGULARLY IRREGULAR + VERY FAST (> 200 bpm) + WPW history or baseline delta wave. QRS morphology varies beat to beat. This is pre-excited AF: the AF impulses are conducting via the accessory pathway rather than (or in addition to) the AV node.

THE TRAP: Administering the ordered diltiazem. Diltiazem blocks the AV node and paradoxically shortens the accessory pathway refractory period, forcing all 350-600 fibrillatory impulses per minute exclusively through the AP, producing ventricular rates > 300 bpm and VF. The same mechanism applies to adenosine, verapamil, digoxin, and IV beta-blockers.

ACTION: HOLD the diltiazem order. Notify the physician immediately that this is pre-excited AF and that diltiazem is absolutely contraindicated. State the correct management: IV procainamide (stable) or immediate unsynchronized defibrillation 200 J (unstable). Document the hold and the communication with rationale.

ABSOLUTE CONTRAINDICATIONS IN PRE-EXCITED AF — MEMORIZE THIS LIST: Adenosine · Verapamil · Diltiazem · Digoxin · IV Beta-blockers. All five block the AV node. In pre-excited AF, blocking the AV node removes the only rate-limiting structure between the fibrillating atria and the ventricles, allowing the accessory pathway to conduct at rates that produce VF. This is a patient safety intervention that the nurse must be prepared to make even before the physician arrives at the bedside.

4.5 Posterior MI — The STEMI with No Elevation

Posterior myocardial infarction is the territory most likely to be missed entirely on the standard 12-lead because no standard electrode faces the posterior wall directly. The posterior MI announces itself with a reciprocal pattern — ST depression and tall R waves in V1-V2 — that can be easily dismissed as 'anterior ischemia' or 'non-specific changes' by a nurse or provider who does not know to look for the posterior pattern.

POSTERIOR MI

LOOKS LIKE: A patient with chest pain whose 12-lead shows ST depression and tall R waves in V1-V2, but no ST elevation anywhere. Provider documents 'no STEMI, possible NSTEMI — serial troponins.'

ECG CLUE: ST depression in V1-V2 (often 2-3 mm) combined with tall, broad, upright R waves in V1-V2 (R > S in V1). These are the RECIPROCAL equivalents of posterior ST elevation and posterior Q waves — the posterior wall's electrical changes appear inverted on the standard precordial leads because those leads are viewing the posterior wall from the opposite side.

THE TRAP: Accepting ST depression in V1-V2 as anterior ischemia or non-specific change without obtaining posterior leads. Posterior MI is a STEMI-equivalent requiring emergent reperfusion — missing it means missing a cath lab activation.

ACTION: Obtain posterior leads V7-V9 immediately. Place electrodes at the left posterior chest: V7 at the posterior axillary line, V8 at the left scapular tip, V9 at the left paraspinal border — all at the same horizontal level as V4-V6. Threshold for posterior MI: ST elevation ≥0.5 mm in ≥2 contiguous posterior leads (lower than the standard precordial threshold, to account for signal attenuation at increased electrode distance). If positive: STEMI protocol activation.

Posterior Lead Placement	Landmark
V7	Left posterior axillary line, at the same horizontal level as V4 (5th intercostal space)
V8	Left scapular tip (at the angle of the scapula), same horizontal level
V9	Left paraspinal border (immediately left of the vertebral column), same horizontal level
Threshold	ST elevation ≥0.5 mm in ≥2 contiguous posterior leads = posterior MI confirmed

4.6 Electrical Alternans — Tamponade Until Echo Proves Otherwise

Electrical alternans in the context of a hemodynamically compromised patient is a cardiac imaging emergency. The pattern — beat-to-beat alternation in QRS amplitude — reflects a large pericardial effusion with the heart physically swinging within the fluid-filled pericardial sac. When combined with the clinical signs of cardiac tamponade, the next step is always bedside echocardiography, not additional laboratory testing or a return to monitoring.

ELECTRICAL ALTERNANS + TAMPONADE

LOOKS LIKE: A patient with dyspnea, hypotension, and JVD whose ECG shows what appears to be 'changing QRS size' on the monitor. The troponin is ordered. Provider plans further workup.

ECG CLUE: Regular alternation of QRS amplitude every other beat — one beat large, the next small, the next large again, throughout the strip. Combined with low voltage in all limb leads (< 5 mm) and sinus tachycardia. The clinical context: hypotension, JVD, muffled heart sounds (Beck's triad), and a history of malignancy, post-cardiac surgery, pericarditis, or chest trauma.

THE TRAP: Ordering troponin and waiting for laboratory results while the patient deteriorates. Cardiac tamponade is a clinical-echocardiographic diagnosis, not a laboratory diagnosis. The troponin does not identify or quantify the effusion. Every minute without pericardiocentesis in true tamponade increases the risk of cardiac arrest from PEA.

ACTION: Bedside echocardiography IMMEDIATELY. Notify the physician of Beck's triad, low voltage, and electrical alternans and specifically request an urgent echo to assess for pericardial effusion with RV/RA collapse. Prepare for emergency pericardiocentesis. Keep the defibrillator at the bedside — tamponade can progress to PEA arrest without warning.

Tamponade Clinical Sign	Description and Significance
Beck's Triad	(1) Hypotension — the pericardial fluid under pressure compresses the ventricles and reduces stroke volume. (2) Jugular venous distension (JVD) — elevated venous pressure from impaired ventricular filling. (3) Muffled heart sounds — the surrounding fluid attenuates the sound transmitted to the chest wall. All three are present in classic acute tamponade; some may be absent in slowly developing effusions.
Pulsus paradoxus	An exaggerated fall in systolic BP (≥ 10 mmHg) during normal inspiration. Reflects the exaggerated interventricular interdependence under pericardial constraint — as the RV fills during inspiration, it bulges into the LV, reducing LV output. Measured with a blood pressure cuff while the patient breathes normally.
Electrical alternans mechanism	The large effusion allows the heart to physically rotate or swing within the pericardial sac with each beat (the 'swinging heart'). The alternating position relative to the fixed surface electrodes produces the alternating QRS amplitude. The amplitude alternation is most prominent in QRS complexes; P waves and T waves may also alternate.

Echo findings confirming tamponade	Right atrial collapse during ventricular systole (earlier, more sensitive). Right ventricular collapse during diastole (more specific for hemodynamic tamponade). These are the definitive signs that distinguish tamponade from simple pericardial effusion without hemodynamic compromise.

4.7 The Six-Pattern Recognition Summary

The following table consolidates all six high-risk patterns from this chapter into a single reference format. The most important column is the last one — the wrong action that is commonly taken when the pattern is not recognized.

Pattern	ECG Clue	Correct Action	Wrong Action to Avoid
Wellens syndrome	Deep symmetric T inversions V2-V3 (pain-free)	Urgent cardiology consult, NPO, prepare for angiography	Stress testing — can trigger massive STEMI
De Winter pattern	Upsloping ST depression + tall peaked T waves V1-V4	STEMI-equivalent activation — call the cath lab	Admit as NSTEMI, wait for troponin
Left main / aVR elevation	Diffuse ST depression ≥6 leads + aVR elevation ≥1 mm	Urgent angiography — same urgency as STEMI	Serial troponins, routine NSTEMI workup
Pre-excited AF	Wide + irregular + > 200 bpm + WPW	Procainamide IV (stable) or defibrillate (unstable)	Adenosine / verapamil / diltiazem → VF

Posterior MI	ST depression + tall R in V1-V2, no elevation	Obtain V7-V9 immediately (≥0.5 mm = STEMI)	Accept as 'anterior ischemia,' miss the activation
Electrical alternans + tamponade	Beat-to-beat QRS amplitude alternation + low voltage	Bedside echo immediately, prepare pericardiocentesi s	Order troponin, wait for lab results

4.8 Communication Framework for High-Risk Pattern Recognition

Recognizing a high-risk pattern is the first half of the job. The second half is communicating it in a way that generates the correct response from the physician, even if the physician has not seen the ECG yet and even if the pattern is one they might not independently recognize under time pressure.

HIGH-RISK PATTERN COMMUNICATION TEMPLATE

Use this template for any of the six patterns in this chapter:

1. Name the pattern: 'I am seeing a [Wellens / de Winter / aVR elevation / pre-excited AF / posterior MI / electrical alternans] pattern on this ECG.'

2. State what it means: 'This indicates [critical proximal LAD stenosis / acute LAD occlusion / left main disease / pre-excited AF with VF risk / posterior STEMI / cardiac tamponade].'

3. State what you need: 'I need [cardiology at the bedside urgently / cath lab activation / procainamide instead of diltiazem / posterior leads obtained / bedside echo immediately].'

4. State what you are holding or doing now: 'I am holding the [diltiazem order / stress test request] until you arrive.' / 'I am obtaining V7-V9 now.'

DOCUMENT EVERY COMMUNICATION: For each of the six patterns, document in the chart: (1) the time the pattern was identified, (2) the exact ECG finding that triggered the concern, (3) the name of the provider notified, (4) the time of notification, (5) the provider's response, and (6) any order held with the rationale. This documentation is both a patient safety record and a professional protection for the nurse who identified the pattern.

BEDSIDE PEARL The consistent theme across all six patterns: the ECG finding does not match the conventional visual expectation for a cardiac emergency. Wellens — no ST elevation, pain-free patient. De Winter — no ST elevation, ST depression instead. Left main — no regional elevation, diffuse depression looks non-specific. Pre-excited AF — the wide irregular tachycardia looks like it could be 'just AF with aberrancy.' Posterior MI — no elevation on the standard leads, only depression. Electrical alternans — the QRS amplitude variation looks like 'the monitor is fluctuating.' The unifying clinical skill is not memorizing patterns. It is resisting the instinct to dismiss a subtle or atypical finding in a patient with a convincing clinical story.

KEY POINTS — CHAPTER 4

Wellens Syndrome

- Deep symmetric T inversion V2-V3 (Type A) or biphasic T waves V2-V3 (Type B) in a pain-free patient = critical proximal LAD stenosis.
- Stress test is ABSOLUTELY CONTRAINDICATED. Urgent angiography is the correct next step. Communicate the pattern by name to the physician.

De Winter Pattern

- Upsloping J-point depression + tall peaked T waves in V1-V4 = LAD occlusion without ST elevation. STEMI-equivalent urgency — activate the cath lab.

Left Main Pattern

- Diffuse ST depression ≥6 leads + ST elevation in aVR ≥1 mm = left main or severe multivessel disease. Urgent angiography, not serial troponin workup.

Pre-Excited AF

- Wide + irregular + > 200 bpm + WPW = pre-excited AF. HOLD adenosine, verapamil, diltiazem, digoxin, and IV beta-blockers. Procainamide (stable) or immediate defibrillation (unstable).

Posterior MI and Electrical Alternans

- ST depression + tall R in V1-V2 = obtain V7-V9 (≥0.5 mm threshold for posterior MI). Do not accept as 'anterior ischemia' without posterior leads.
- Electrical alternans + Beck's triad + low voltage = tamponade. Bedside echo immediately. Prepare for pericardiocentesis. Troponin does not diagnose or quantify pericardial effusion.

REMEMBER THIS

- ✓ All six patterns share one feature: they look less alarming than they are. The ECG finding that identifies a critical LAD stenosis (Wellens), an active LAD occlusion (de Winter), left main disease (aVR elevation), VF-triggering AF (pre-excited), a missed STEMI (posterior MI), or impending PEA arrest (tamponade) does not produce the visual drama of a classic STEMI with 4 mm of ST elevation across six leads. The clinical skill is recognizing the subtle finding and acting on it at the same speed as a classic STEMI.
- ✓ For pre-excited AF: the contraindication list must be automatic — adenosine, verapamil, diltiazem, digoxin, and IV beta-blockers. All five produce the same mechanism (AV node blockade → all AF impulses through the AP → VF), and the error can occur faster than the physician can be reached by phone. The nurse who recognizes the pattern and holds the medication order is the last safety check before a preventable VF.
- ✓ For Wellens syndrome: the most important action is a communication action, not a medication action. The patient may look completely well. The physician may not be at the bedside. The stress test order may already be written. The

nurse's role is to name the pattern, state its significance, and hold any stress test or discharge orders until a physician has reviewed the ECG at the bedside. This is the definition of advocacy in high-risk ECG recognition.

ICU Telemetry — Recognition to Escalation

Continuous monitoring: what to act on vs what to document

ICU NURSING · RAPID RESPONSE · NCLEX

Continuous cardiac monitoring in the ICU produces an enormous volume of data — hundreds of rhythm strips, thousands of alarm triggers, and a continuous ST segment trend — across every shift. The clinical skill this chapter addresses is not pattern recognition in isolation. It is the judgment to distinguish findings that require immediate action from findings that require documentation, findings that require a provider call from findings that require a medication hold, and findings that are artifact from findings that are real.

The sections that follow build a structured approach to ICU telemetry that is neither hyper-reactive (acting on every alarm) nor under-reactive (silencing alarms without assessment). Both failure modes produce patient harm.

5.1 Telemetry Alarm Fatigue — The Core Problem

Alarm fatigue is the most well-documented patient safety issue in modern cardiac monitoring. Studies consistently show that on a busy ICU or telemetry unit, more than 85% of monitor alarms are clinically insignificant — false alarms from artifact, from normal physiological variation, or from alarm thresholds that are not individualized to the patient. When virtually every alarm is non-actionable, clinicians begin responding more slowly to alarms, or stop responding systematically at all.

The consequences are predictable: the infrequent but critical alarm — the one that signals VT, VF, complete AV block, or a dynamic ST change in a STEMI patient — is delayed in its response. Alarm fatigue has been directly implicated in preventable patient deaths in published root cause analyses. Addressing it is not a technology problem — it is a clinical nursing practice problem.

Alarm Fatigue Contributor	Nursing Practice Solution
Default alarm thresholds not individualized	Set HR high and low limits to patient-appropriate ranges: a marathon runner with a resting HR of 48 bpm should not have a 60 bpm low-HR alarm. A patient with known AF should have an irregular-rhythm alarm disabled if AF is their documented baseline.
Poor electrode contact producing false alarms	Skin preparation: clip hair, clean with soap and water or alcohol wipe, allow to dry fully before electrode placement. Replace electrodes every 24 hours and immediately if the impedance alarm fires. Poor skin prep is the single most preventable source of artifact alarms.
Alarm sounds desensitizing nursing response	Use escalating alarm tiers (low-priority visual-only, medium-priority audio, high-priority persistent audio) so that the audio environment prioritizes life-threatening alarms. Document alarm threshold settings at the start of each shift and when they are changed.
No clear threshold for action vs documentation	Establish and follow a tiered response protocol (Section 5.2). Every alarm is assessed; the response level is determined by the clinical finding, not by a reflexive accept/silence.

5.2 Tiered Response Protocol — Act vs Document vs Silence

A tiered response protocol assigns a predetermined response level to each category of alarm finding, removing the uncertainty of 'what should I do with this?' from each individual decision. The following three tiers cover the full range of ICU telemetry findings.

Tier	Finding Category	Response

1 ACT NOW	VF, VT > 30 seconds, complete AV block with wide escape, sustained bradycardia < 30 bpm with hemodynamic compromise, pulseless rhythm, dynamic ST change in a known STEMI patient	Immediate bedside assessment. Activate the appropriate response (ACLS, RRT, or Code Blue depending on the rhythm and the patient's hemodynamic status). Do not silence the alarm; do not wait to confirm remotely.
2 ASSESS AND NOTIFY	New AF or atrial flutter, non-sustained VT (< 30 s), Mobitz II, new complete AV block with narrow escape, QTc prolonging above 0.50 s, new ST depression or elevation on CSTM trend, significant rate change (tachycardia > 130 or bradycardia < 45 in a previously stable patient)	Bedside assessment within 5 minutes. Vital signs, clinical assessment. Notify provider with SBAR. Document the finding, assessment, and notification time. Prepare for potential intervention.
3 DOCUMENT	Known baseline rhythm variant (e.g., chronic AF with rate in the monitored range, benign sinus arrhythmia, known ectopy within expected frequency), single PVC on a patient not on a post-MI protocol, transient rate alarm that self-resolved within 30 seconds, artifact identified and corrected	Document the alarm, the assessment, and the conclusion. Correct artifact sources (reposition lead, improve electrode contact). Update alarm threshold if appropriate. No provider notification required unless clinical change.

5.3 Continuous ST-Segment Monitoring (CSTM)

Continuous ST-segment monitoring is a standard-of-care recommendation for patients in the first 24-72 hours after ACS, post-cardiac surgery, and in any patient at high risk for ischemia in the ICU. It provides a real-time ST trend that no single-time-point 12-lead can offer — it detects dynamic changes over hours that would be invisible on the standard spot-check ECG schedule.

CSTM Lead Selection

- The optimal monitoring leads for CSTM depend on the territory at risk. For anterior STEMI patients or LAD territory: leads V1-V3 provide the best anterior sensitivity. For inferior STEMI patients or RCA territory: Lead II (or aVF if available) provides the best inferior sensitivity.
- Most bedside monitors provide CSTM in two to three simultaneous leads. Select leads that cover both the territory at risk (based on the patient's diagnosis) and the rhythm monitoring lead (typically lead II for P wave visibility).
- Establish the CSTM baseline at the time of patient admission or immediately after any acute intervention (PCI, cardioversion, thrombolytics). The baseline is the reference against which all trend changes are measured.

CSTM Threshold for Notification

- A change from the established CSTM baseline of ≥1 mm in any monitored lead, sustained for ≥60 seconds, is the standard threshold for provider notification in most institutional CSTM protocols.
- A change of ≥2 mm sustained for ≥60 seconds represents a higher-urgency threshold requiring more immediate response, particularly in the first 24 hours post-ACS.
- Dynamic ST changes that track with changes in patient symptoms (increasing chest pain correlating with worsening ST trend) are more clinically significant than isolated asymptomatic ST changes of the same magnitude.

CSTM SETUP CHECKLIST AT PATIENT ADMISSION:

1. Confirm the monitor is set to display CSTM trend (not just a rhythm channel). Verify the monitoring leads selected match the territory at risk for this patient.
2. Establish and document the baseline ST measurement in each monitored lead immediately after patient stabilization or after any acute intervention.
3. Set CSTM alarm thresholds: low-urgency alert at ≥1 mm change from baseline; high-urgency alert at ≥2 mm change from baseline. Document the thresholds in the patient chart.
4. Confirm CSTM alarm is active and audible (not silenced or downgraded to visual-only). CSTM alarm silence should never be the default state for an acute ICU patient.
5. Document the initial CSTM setup: leads selected, baseline values, alarm thresholds, and time of setup. This documentation allows any nurse inheriting the patient to understand the monitoring parameters in use.

5.4 QTc Monitoring in the ICU

QTc prolongation is one of the most common preventable drug-related arrhythmia risks in the ICU. The ICU environment concentrates multiple QTc-prolonging factors simultaneously — multiple QTc-prolonging medications, electrolyte disorders (hypokalemia, hypomagnesemia), bradycardia, and baseline cardiac disease — making QTc monitoring both more important and more complex than in a general ward.

QTc Monitoring Scenario	Nursing Action
QTc > 0.44 s (women) or > 0.43 s (men) at baseline ICU admission	Document baseline QTc. Review all medications for QTc-prolonging agents. Flag to prescribing team. Correct electrolytes: target K^+ ≥4.0 mEq/L and Mg^{2+} ≥2.0 mEq/L.
QTc 0.44–0.50 s with QTc-prolonging drug newly started	Obtain a 12-lead ECG 4-6 hours after each dose escalation. Notify provider of QTc value. Ensure electrolyte repletion is ordered. Consider requesting an alternative agent with lower QTc risk if available.

QTc > 0.50 s	Notify provider immediately. QTc ≥ 0.50 s significantly increases torsades de pointes risk. Provider review of all QTc-prolonging medications is required. Consider holding the most recently added agent while the team reviews. Ensure defibrillator is immediately available at the bedside.
New polymorphic VT (torsades) in a patient with prolonged QTc	Immediate bedside assessment. IV magnesium sulfate 2 g IV over 5-15 minutes (first-line). Notify provider urgently. Hold ALL QTc-prolonging medications. Do NOT give amiodarone (further prolongs QT). Prepare for cardioversion if torsades is sustained.
Sudden QTc shortening (QTc < 0.35 s)	Obtain 12-lead ECG and check calcium level. Hypercalcemia shortens the QT. Sudden QTc shortening in a previously normal-QT patient may also reflect electrolyte abnormality or, rarely, congenital short QT syndrome.

> **COMMON ICU QTc-PROLONGING DRUGS:** Antibiotics (azithromycin, ciprofloxacin, fluconazole), antipsychotics (haloperidol, quetiapine), antiemetics (ondansetron, promethazine), antiarrhythmics (amiodarone, sotalol, dofetilide), methadone, some antivirals. This list is not exhaustive. When in doubt, check the patient's medication list against a QTc risk resource (such as CredibleMeds / Arizona CERT) before adding any new agent to a patient with a borderline or prolonged baseline QTc.

5.5 Artifact vs Arrhythmia in the ICU

ICU patients generate more monitoring artifact than general ward patients because of their condition: continuous movement from restlessness, shivering, or positioning changes; multiple devices attached to the same patient (ventilator, IV pumps, bed); and frequent interventions that disrupt electrode contact. Distinguishing true arrhythmia from artifact is a core ICU monitoring skill.

Artifact Type	ECG Appearance	Distinguishing from True Arrhythmia

Motion artifact (patient movement)	Irregular chaotic waveform, may resemble VF or VT. Typically has some underlying organized QRS complexes visible at the beginning or end of the artifact burst.	Correlates temporally with patient movement (shivering, repositioning, procedure). The patient is conscious and responsive. The artifact starts and stops abruptly. True VF or VT in an awake patient without symptoms is rare.
60-Hz electrical interference	Regular sinusoidal waveform at 60 cycles per second superimposed on the baseline. May appear as a uniformly thickened baseline.	Regular, perfectly sinusoidal, constant amplitude — true arrhythmias are not perfectly regular. Check for nearby electrical equipment. Ground the patient cable. Try a different lead.
Poor electrode contact	Flat baseline in one lead, intermittent signal, large baseline wander. May appear as asystole in the affected lead.	Check the specific lead cable connection and electrode adherence. A flat line in one lead with normal signals in other leads = electrode problem, not asystole. Asystole is global — confirmed in multiple leads simultaneously.
Ventilator-related baseline wander	Rhythmic, slow oscillation of the baseline at the respiratory rate of the ventilator.	The wander follows the ventilator rate exactly. Slow, regular, sinusoidal at a rate much lower than the heart rate. True ST elevation or depression is not rhythmically synchronous with the ventilator.

IV pump interference	Intermittent spike or burst artifact, often at regular intervals corresponding to pump cycles.	Compare the timing of the artifact to the IV pump cycle. Reposition the pump power supply away from the monitor if possible. Check grounding.

THE MOST DANGEROUS ARTIFACT ERROR: Mistaking motion artifact for VF and performing an unnecessary defibrillation on an awake patient. Always assess the patient clinically before defibrillating: is the patient unresponsive? Is there no pulse? If the patient is awake and talking, the chaotic waveform is artifact. A 10-second clinical assessment before defibrillation prevents this error.

5.6 Mechanical Ventilation and ECG

Positive pressure ventilation changes the thoracic pressure and cardiac position with each breath, producing ECG changes that are purely physiological and not indicative of any primary cardiac pathology. Understanding these expected ventilator-related ECG changes prevents false alarms and inappropriate interventions.

- Baseline wander: the most common ventilator-related ECG finding. Each positive-pressure breath changes the electrical axis of the heart slightly as the lungs inflate, producing a rhythmic oscillation of the ECG baseline at the ventilator rate. This is most visible in the limb leads and should not be mistaken for ST elevation or depression.
- QRS axis variation: in patients on high PEEP (positive end-expiratory pressure), the sustained increase in intrathoracic pressure can produce a detectable shift in the mean QRS axis compared to the patient's spontaneous-breathing baseline.
- Sinus arrhythmia pattern: some patients show respiratory-phase variation in the R-R interval that corresponds to the ventilator cycle. This is a normal phenomenon (respiratory sinus arrhythmia) and should not be mistaken for an irregular rhythm or AF in a patient with a history of AF.

- ST changes with ventilator disconnection: if a patient is briefly disconnected from the ventilator for suctioning or during weaning trials, ST changes can appear from the acute change in intrathoracic pressure and cardiac preload. Document the ventilator status at the time of any ST change in a mechanically ventilated patient.

5.7 Pacemaker Monitoring in the Post-Implant Period

The first 24-72 hours after pacemaker implantation are the highest-risk period for device malfunction, specifically lead displacement — the period before fibrous tissue secures the leads in place. ICU and step-down nurses caring for post-implant patients must be familiar with the expected appearance of paced rhythms and the three categories of malfunction that can occur in this window.

Malfunction	ECG Appearance	Immediate Action
Failure to capture	Pacing spikes visible at expected intervals, but no P wave (atrial lead) or QRS complex (ventricular lead) follows the spike.	Assess hemodynamics immediately. Notify provider urgently. If pacemaker-dependent patient: prepare TCP. Chest X-ray to assess lead position. Device interrogation required.
Failure to sense (undersensing)	Pacing spikes appear during the patient's intrinsic rhythm — competitive pacing. Risk of R-on-T if ventricular lead fires on the T wave of a native beat.	Defibrillator to bedside immediately (R-on-T risk). Notify provider urgently. Do NOT apply magnet (this converts to asynchronous pacing, which worsens R-on-T risk in undersensing). Device interrogation to increase sensing sensitivity.

Failure to pace (failure to output)	No pacing spikes appear when the rate falls below the set minimum. Rate drops to the patient's intrinsic or escape rate.	If pacemaker-dependent : prepare TCP immediately. Notify provider urgently. Check battery status indicator. Chest X-ray. Device interrogation. Possible generator replacement required.

POST-IMPLANT ACTIVITY RESTRICTIONS: The most common cause of early post-implant failure to capture is lead displacement from premature ipsilateral arm elevation or vigorous ipsilateral shoulder movement. Nursing instructions for post-implant patients: no lifting the arm on the implant side above shoulder level, no vigorous reaching, no sleeping on the implant side for the first 4-6 weeks. Document patient education and any new symptoms (palpitations, dizziness, or pacing sensations) at each assessment.

5.8 ICU Telemetry Documentation Standards

Documentation in the ICU telemetry setting serves three functions: it creates a clinical record for continuity of care, it provides evidence of nursing assessment and response for medicolegal purposes, and it creates the data trail needed for quality improvement and root cause analysis when adverse events occur. The following documentation standards apply to all significant telemetry findings in the ICU.

REQUIRED DOCUMENTATION ELEMENTS FOR SIGNIFICANT ICU TELEMETRY FINDINGS:

1. Time of finding identification: the exact time the rhythm change or alarm was first noted on the monitor display.

2. Description of the finding: rate, rhythm name, QRS width, any ST change (lead, magnitude, direction), or alarm type.

3. Clinical assessment at the time of the finding: patient's level of consciousness, vital signs (HR, BP, SpO_2, RR), symptoms reported, and whether the finding is new or a known baseline.

4. Tier classification: whether the finding was classified as Tier 1 (Act Now), Tier 2 (Assess and Notify), or Tier 3 (Document), and the rationale.

5. Provider notification: name of provider notified, method of communication (phone, bedside), time of notification, and provider's verbal response.
6. Action taken: specific intervention (medication administered, cardioversion performed, TCP applied, defibrillator to bedside) or watchful waiting, with the rationale for the chosen response.
7. Patient response: vital sign trend after intervention, rhythm status on follow-up assessment (time and finding).
8. CSTM status (if applicable): current CSTM trend value in monitored leads at the time of any ST-related finding, and comparison to the documented baseline.

BEDSIDE PEARL The ICU telemetry discipline that separates effective from ineffective monitoring: every alarm is assessed at the bedside before it is silenced. Not every alarm requires an intervention, a provider call, or even a chart note beyond the assessment — but every alarm requires a human clinical assessment. The nurse who walks to the bedside, checks the patient, confirms the finding is artifact or a known baseline variant, and documents the assessment has done exactly the right thing. The nurse who silences the alarm from the workstation without assessment has eliminated the safety check that exists between an ignored alarm and a patient harm event.

KEY POINTS — CHAPTER 5

Alarm Fatigue and Tiered Response

- Individualize alarm thresholds at the start of every shift. A patient with chronic AF should not have an irregular-rhythm alarm active. A patient with a resting HR of 48 bpm should not have a 60 bpm low-HR alarm.
- Tier 1 (Act Now): VF, sustained VT, complete AV block with wide escape, hemodynamic compromise from brady/tachy. Tier 2 (Assess and Notify): new AF, non-sustained VT, QTc > 0.50, new ST change. Tier 3 (Document): known baseline variants, transient self-resolving alarms, artifact identified and corrected.

CSTM and QTc

- CSTM: establish baseline immediately on admission; set ≥1 mm and ≥2 mm thresholds; lead selection should cover territory at risk. Notify provider for any sustained ≥1 mm change from baseline.
- QTc > 0.50 s = notify provider immediately, review all QTc-prolonging drugs, ensure K^+ ≥4.0 and Mg^{2+} ≥2.0, defibrillator at bedside. Never give amiodarone for torsades — it further prolongs QT.

Artifact and Post-Implant Monitoring

- Motion artifact mimics VF but the patient is awake and responsive. Always assess the patient clinically before defibrillating. A 10-second assessment prevents unnecessary shocks.
- Ventilator-related ECG changes (baseline wander, respiratory sinus arrhythmia) are physiological and expected. Document ventilator status at the time of any ST change in a ventilated patient.
- Post-implant malfunction: failure to capture (spikes present, no QRS) vs failure to sense (competitive pacing, R-on-T risk — defibrillator to bedside) vs failure to output (no spikes — prepare TCP if pacemaker-dependent).

REMEMBER THIS

✓ Every alarm is assessed at the bedside before it is silenced — this is the non-negotiable standard that prevents alarm fatigue from becoming patient harm. The assessment may take 30 seconds and conclude that the finding is artifact or a known baseline variant. That is a clinically valid outcome. Silencing an alarm from the workstation without bedside assessment removes the human safety check from the monitoring chain.

✓ QTc > 0.50 s in an ICU patient requires immediate action: provider notification, medication review, electrolyte correction, and a defibrillator at the bedside. The ICU medication list is the most likely cause — antibiotics, antipsychotics, antiemetics, and antiarrhythmics all carry QTc risk, and their combined effect is additive. Never add a new QTc-prolonging agent to a patient with a baseline QTc > 0.44 s without checking the cumulative QTc risk.

✓ The three post-implant pacemaker malfunctions are distinguished by whether spikes are present and whether they capture: spikes present but no QRS = failure to capture (lead displacement, check X-ray); spikes on native beats = failure to sense (R-on-T risk, defibrillator to bedside, do not apply magnet); no spikes when rate falls below set minimum = failure to output (battery or lead fracture, prepare TCP if pacemaker-dependent).

Post-Cardiac Surgery ECG Changes

What is expected vs what is dangerous after open heart surgery

ICU NURSING · CARDIAC SURGERY · NCLEX

The cardiac surgery ICU presents a monitoring challenge unique in all of critical care: the patient arrives with ECG changes that would be alarming in any other context and are entirely expected in this one. Sinus tachycardia, nonspecific ST-T changes, low voltage, new bundle branch blocks, and temporary pacing dependency are all routine post-operative findings that should not trigger a STEMI workup or emergency cardiology call. The clinical skill is knowing which findings fall into the expected category — and which fall into the small but critical group that indicate a genuine post-operative complication requiring urgent intervention.

This chapter organizes post-cardiac surgery ECG findings into two tracks: expected and dangerous. Every finding is presented in the context of the specific surgical procedure that most commonly produces it, with the clinical actions appropriate to each.

6.1 Expected Post-Operative ECG Changes

The following ECG findings are expected consequences of the physiological effects of general anesthesia, cardiopulmonary bypass, cardiac manipulation, pericardiotomy, and the metabolic derangements of major surgery. Their presence on the immediate post-operative ECG should be documented and monitored but does not require emergent intervention.

ECG Finding	Mechanism	Expected Duration / Action

Sinus tachycardia (HR 90-120 bpm)	Catecholamine surge from surgery, pain, anesthesia emergence, hypovolemia, fever, anemia — all are common in the first 12-24 post-op hours.	Typically resolves within 24-48 hours as the patient stabilizes. If HR persists > 120 bpm: assess for hypovolemia, pain, fever, bleeding, anemia, or tamponade. Sinus tachycardia is always secondary — treat the cause.
Nonspecific ST-T changes	Cardiac manipulation during surgery, pericardiotomy, myocardial stunning from bypass, and the metabolic effects of cardioplegia all alter repolarization nonspecifically.	Expected for the first 24-72 hours. Stable, non-dynamic changes in a hemodynamically stable patient require documentation, not urgent investigation. Dynamic changes or new regional patterns require urgent assessment (see Section 6.6).
Low voltage in limb leads (QRS < 5 mm)	Pericardial and mediastinal fluid accumulation after cardiac surgery. May also reflect anasarca (generalized fluid overload) in bypass patients.	Monitor for worsening low voltage, electrical alternans, or JVD — these indicate effusion with tamponade physiology (Section 6.6). Stable low voltage without hemodynamic compromise: monitor with serial echocardiography.
PR prolongation (first-degree AV block)	Edema of the AV nodal tissue from surgical manipulation or cardioplegia. Common after aortic or mitral valve surgery.	Usually resolves within days to weeks. Document and monitor. No action required unless PR extends > 0.24 s or progresses to higher-degree block.

Rate-dependent right bundle branch block	Edema of the right bundle branch from surgical manipulation or bypass. More common after procedures near the interventricular septum.	Often resolves within days. Document QRS width serially. If RBBB persists at discharge: cardiology follow-up for pacemaker consideration if combined with symptoms.

6.2 Post-Operative Atrial Fibrillation

Post-operative AF is the most common arrhythmia complication after cardiac surgery, occurring in 20-40% of patients after CABG and up to 50% after combined CABG-valve procedures. It typically occurs in the first 2-4 days after surgery, with peak incidence on post-operative day 2. Its presence is expected enough that many cardiac surgery programs have standing orders for its management.

Why Post-Op AF Occurs

- Inflammation: surgery and cardiopulmonary bypass produce a systemic inflammatory response that increases atrial irritability.
- Electrolyte derangements: hypokalemia and hypomagnesemia from bypass-related diuresis and fluid shifts lower the threshold for atrial arrhythmias.
- Sympathetic activation: catecholamine surge from surgery and pain increases automaticity throughout the atrium.
- Atrial stretch: volume loading during bypass and post-operative fluid resuscitation increases atrial wall tension.

Management Framework

Clinical Status	Management

Hemodynamically STABLE post-op AF	Rate control first: IV metoprolol or IV diltiazem (diltiazem is appropriate here because the rhythm is AF, not VT, and the patient does not have WPW). Target ventricular rate < 110 bpm at rest. Correct electrolytes: replete K^+ to ≥4.0 mEq/L and Mg^{2+} to ≥2.0 mEq/L — this alone restores sinus rhythm in a significant proportion of post-op AF. Anticoagulation: most post-op AF patients require anticoagulation; discuss timing with the surgical team given the recent sternotomy (bleeding risk vs stroke risk balance).
Hemodynamically UNSTABLE post-op AF (BP < 90, acute pulmonary edema, ischemia)	Synchronized cardioversion: 120-200 J biphasic synchronized. Post-op patients who develop hemodynamically significant AF in the first 48 hours after surgery often convert with cardioversion and stay in sinus rhythm once the inciting physiological insults resolve. Amiodarone 150 mg IV over 10 minutes can be given concurrently as a rhythm-control adjunct and to reduce recurrence post-cardioversion.
Recurrent or persistent post-op AF (> 48-72 hours)	Cardiology consultation for rhythm vs rate control decision. If AF persists > 48 hours without anticoagulation: TEE to exclude left atrial thrombus before cardioversion. Long-term anticoagulation per CHA_2DS_2-VASc scoring.

ELECTROLYTE REPLETION FIRST: Before any antiarrhythmic drug for post-op AF, confirm and correct K^+ and Mg^{2+}. Bypass-related diuresis commonly produces hypokalemia and hypomagnesemia that independently sustain AF. A patient with K^+ 3.1 and Mg^{2+} 1.3 who is cardioverted without electrolyte correction will frequently revert to AF within hours. Replace to target levels first, then reassess the rhythm.

6.3 Postpericardiotomy Syndrome

Postpericardiotomy syndrome is an inflammatory pericarditis that develops 2-6 weeks after any cardiac surgery involving pericardiotomy (cutting the pericardium). It occurs in approximately 10-40% of post-cardiac surgery patients and presents with the classic four-stage ECG changes of acute pericarditis (Book 3, Chapter 10) in a patient who had cardiac surgery weeks before. Recognizing it prevents both a missed diagnosis and an unnecessary workup for recurrent ischemia.

Feature	Details
Timing	2-6 weeks after cardiac surgery. This is later than the immediate post-op period and later than the expected sinus tachycardia and nonspecific ST changes of the first 48-72 hours.
ECG findings	Classic Stage 1 pericarditis: diffuse concave ST elevation across most of the 12-lead, PR segment depression in most leads, PR elevation in aVR, NO reciprocal ST depression. The same ECG differentiating features from STEMI that were covered in Book 3 Chapter 10 apply here.
Clinical features	Fever, pleuritic chest pain (worse lying flat, improved sitting forward), pericardial friction rub on auscultation, elevated ESR and CRP.
Distinguishing from post-op MI	Postpericardiotomy: diffuse concave elevation, PR depression, no reciprocal changes, systemic inflammatory signs. Post-op MI (graft failure): regional convex elevation with reciprocal depression in the expected mirror-image leads, troponin rise, hemodynamic compromise.
Treatment	NSAIDs (ibuprofen 600-800 mg three times daily) + colchicine 0.5 mg twice daily for 3 months. Corticosteroids are reserved for refractory cases. Note: corticosteroids increase the risk of recurrence in pericarditis and impair surgical wound healing in the post-op period — they should be avoided as first-line treatment.

6.4 Conduction Changes After Cardiac Surgery

New conduction abnormalities are common after cardiac surgery, particularly procedures that involve the interventricular septum, the tricuspid valve annulus (close to the AV node), or the aortic valve (which is anatomically adjacent to the left bundle branch and the AV node). Most are transient, but some persist and require long-term follow-up.

Conduction Change	Most Common Surgical Cause	Clinical Significance
New RBBB	VSD repair, CABG with right coronary territory involvement, aortic valve replacement (AVR). The right bundle branch runs along the right ventricular septum near the surgical field for many of these procedures.	Usually benign in isolation if the patient is hemodynamically stable. Monitor for progression to complete AV block (bifascicular RBBB + LAFB pattern or RBBB + first-degree AV block increases pacemaker risk). Cardiology follow-up if persistent at discharge.
New LBBB	Aortic valve replacement (AVR) — the left bundle branch runs immediately below the aortic valve annulus. New LBBB after AVR occurs in 3-8% of patients.	More concerning than isolated RBBB: if symptomatic, obtain echocardiogram to exclude cardiac resynchronization need. New LBBB also complicates future ischemia evaluation (Sgarbossa criteria will be required for any future chest pain ECG).

Complete AV block (immediate post-op)	AVR, mitral valve replacement/repair, VSD closure, or any procedure with direct suturing near the AV node. The AV node sits at the apex of the triangle of Koch in the right atrium, immediately adjacent to the tricuspid valve and the mitral annulus.	Temporary epicardial pacing wires are routinely placed during cardiac surgery precisely for this reason. If complete AV block persists > 5-7 days after surgery and is symptomatic: permanent pacemaker implantation is a Class I indication.
Trifascicular block (RBBB + LAFB + prolonged PR)	CABG or valve surgery with combined conduction system involvement.	High pacemaker risk, particularly if syncope occurs. Class I pacemaker indication for symptomatic trifascicular block post-surgery (consistent with the general trifascicular block criteria from Book 2).

6.5 Temporary Epicardial Pacing Wires

Temporary epicardial pacing wires are placed on the surface of the heart (on the right atrium and right ventricle) during virtually all open-heart surgeries as a precautionary measure against post-operative bradycardia and conduction disturbance. They are one of the most ICU-specific devices the cardiac surgery nurse manages. Their presence, use, and removal each require specific nursing knowledge that is unique to the cardiac surgery setting.

Normal Epicardial Pacing Wire Appearance on ECG

- Pacing spikes may appear in the ECG or they may not, depending on whether the pacemaker is active (patient's intrinsic rate below the set minimum) or inhibited (patient's intrinsic rate above the set minimum).
- Ventricular epicardial pacing: produces a wide LBBB-morphology QRS after each spike (same as any

ventricular pacing — right ventricular activation first). Discordant secondary ST-T changes are expected (Book 2, Chapter 10; Book 4, Section 7).

- Atrial epicardial pacing: produces a pacing spike followed by a normal-appearing QRS (atrial pacing, normal AV conduction). The P wave may or may not be visible depending on the surface electrode orientation.
- Dual-chamber epicardial pacing (atrial + ventricular leads active): atrial spike then ventricular spike, with the same dual-chamber appearance as a permanent DDD pacemaker.

Troubleshooting Epicardial Pacing Wires

Problem	ECG Finding	Action
Failure to capture	Spikes present, no P or QRS follows. May manifest as rate dropping below set minimum in pacemaker-dependent patient.	Increase output (mA) in small increments until capture is restored. Check wire connections. Notify surgeon if capture cannot be restored at maximum safe output.
Failure to sense	Competitive pacing — spikes appear during intrinsic beats. R-on-T risk if ventricular wire fires on a native T wave.	Increase sensing sensitivity on the pacemaker box. Defibrillator to bedside. Notify surgeon. Do NOT simply increase output — this does not address sensing.
Wire displacement or migration	Capture threshold rises progressively over the first 24-48 hours despite increasing output, or complete loss of capture suddenly.	Notify surgeon immediately. May require repositioning. Prepare for TCP as a bridge if the patient is pacemaker-dependent.

Safe removal timing	Wires are typically removed on post-operative day 3-5, once the risk of the initial conduction complications has passed and no pacing dependency has been identified.	The removal of epicardial pacing wires carries a small but real risk of pericardial tamponade from bleeding at the insertion site. Monitor the patient closely for 30-60 minutes after removal: assess BP, HR, and perform a clinical exam for signs of tamponade. Have a defibrillator and echo capability immediately available.

EPICARDIAL WIRE REMOVAL RISK: Cardiac tamponade from pericardial bleeding is a rare but life-threatening complication of epicardial wire removal. It can develop rapidly — within minutes of removal or up to several hours later. Any patient who develops hypotension, JVD, or hemodynamic compromise within 4-6 hours of epicardial wire removal requires immediate bedside echocardiography to exclude tamponade. This clinical pearl should be part of every cardiac surgery nursing handoff when wire removal is planned or has recently occurred.

6.6 Post-Operative Acute MI Recognition

Perioperative myocardial infarction from graft failure or perioperative coronary event occurs in approximately 2-5% of CABG patients and is one of the most serious post-operative complications. Because the post-operative ECG baseline is already abnormal (nonspecific ST-T changes, possible new BBB, pacing dependency), recognizing a superimposed acute MI requires a higher level of vigilance and a lower threshold for investigation than in a non-surgical patient.

POST-OP MI RECOGNITION PROTOCOL — ASSESS ALL FOUR TRIGGERS:

1. New regional ST changes: new ST elevation confined to a specific coronary territory (not diffuse) with or without reciprocal depression, appearing NEW or WORSENED compared to the initial post-op baseline ECG. This requires direct comparison of the current tracing to the admission post-op ECG.

2. Dynamic ST change on CSTM trend: a ≥1 mm change from the established CSTM baseline in a monitored lead, sustained for > 60 seconds, particularly in the first 24 hours after surgery when graft occlusion risk is highest.

3. Hemodynamic deterioration without other explanation: new hypotension, new rhythm disturbances, or new signs of heart failure in the post-op period that are not explained by hypovolemia, bleeding, tamponade, or anesthesia effects.

4. Troponin trend: a significant troponin rise above the expected post-cardiac surgery troponin elevation. Note: all cardiac surgery patients have elevated troponin from myocardial manipulation and CPB — the post-op troponin baseline is higher than in non-surgical patients. A troponin that continues to rise instead of plateauing and declining by 24-48 hours, or that rises dramatically above the institutional post-op baseline range, is concerning for perioperative MI.

TROPONIN AFTER CARDIAC SURGERY: All patients who undergo cardiopulmonary bypass will have elevated troponin — this is expected from myocardial manipulation, cardioplegia, and bypass ischemia-reperfusion. The baseline post-op troponin elevation is not diagnostic of MI. What IS concerning: a troponin that keeps rising beyond 24-48 hours instead of declining, or a troponin value that far exceeds the expected post-op range for the procedure performed. Cardiology consultation should set the threshold for the specific procedure.

6.7 Electrolyte Effects After Cardiopulmonary Bypass

Cardiopulmonary bypass (CPB) produces predictable and clinically important electrolyte derangements that directly affect the ECG and arrhythmia risk in the post-operative period. Understanding the mechanism of each derangement allows the ICU nurse to anticipate ECG changes and act on them before they produce clinical consequences.

Electrolyte	Post-Bypass Trend	ECG Effect and Clinical Action
Potassium (K^+)	Falls — diuresis from CPB-primed fluid, hypothermia-related cellular shifts, and loop diuretics in the post-op period all cause K^+ loss.	Hypokalemia: flat T waves, prominent U waves, QTU prolongation → torsades risk. Target K^+ ≥4.0 mEq/L in all post-cardiac surgery patients. Aggressive IV replacement via central line. Oral KCl once tolerating oral intake.
Magnesium (Mg^{2+})	Falls — bypass circuit dilution and diuresis. Often falls in parallel with potassium.	Hypomagnesemia independently prolongs QT and sustains AF. Target Mg^{2+} ≥2.0 mEq/L. IV magnesium sulfate 2 g over 30-60 min, repeat as needed. Cannot effectively replete K^+ without first addressing Mg^{2+} (Na-K ATPase requires magnesium as a cofactor).
Calcium (Ca^{2+})	Falls — citrate in transfused blood products chelates ionized calcium. Most significant after massive transfusion protocols.	Hypocalcemia: QT prolongation. Severe: cardiac contractility depression, hypotension. IV calcium gluconate 1 g IV over 10-15 min for symptomatic hypocalcemia or ionized Ca^{2+} < 1.0 mmol/L. Monitor ionized calcium (not total calcium) in the post-bypass setting.
Glucose	Rises — CPB, stress response, and cardioplegia solutions (some are glucose-based) all elevate blood glucose, particularly in diabetic patients.	Hyperglycemia increases infection risk and is associated with worse neurological outcomes post-bypass. Target glucose 140-180 mg/dL with insulin infusion per institutional protocol. Extreme hyperglycemia can contribute to osmotic diuresis, worsening hypokalemia.

6.8 The Post-Op ECG Interpretation Framework

Every ECG obtained in the post-cardiac surgery ICU should be interpreted with the following framework, applied in order. The framework prevents both over-investigation (treating expected post-op changes as emergencies) and under-investigation (dismissing dangerous findings as expected changes).

POST-CARDIAC SURGERY ECG INTERPRETATION FRAMEWORK:

1. Compare to the admission post-op baseline ECG. Is any finding NEW or CHANGED from the initial post-op tracing? If YES: it requires specific explanation. If NO and the patient is hemodynamically stable: document as stable post-op ECG findings.

2. Check for regional ST changes. Are any ST changes confined to a specific coronary territory, with reciprocal depression in the mirror-image leads? If YES: concern for post-op MI. Obtain serial ECG, troponin trend, notify surgeon and cardiology.

3. Check for pericarditis pattern. Is there diffuse concave elevation + PR depression + NO reciprocal depression, 2-6 weeks post-op? If YES: consider postpericardiotomy syndrome. Treat with NSAIDs + colchicine.

4. Check the rhythm. Any new AF, new AV block, or new bundle branch block that was not present on the initial post-op ECG requires documentation, provider notification, and management per the protocols in this chapter.

5. Check low voltage trend. Is the low voltage worse than at admission? Worsening low voltage + JVD or hemodynamic instability = bedside echocardiography for tamponade.

6. Check QTc. With multiple electrolyte derangements, multiple QTc-prolonging drugs, and underlying cardiac disease, QTc > 0.50 s is more common in the post-cardiac surgery patient than in the general ICU. Notify provider, correct electrolytes, review medications.

BEDSIDE PEARL The single most important habit in post-cardiac surgery ECG monitoring: always compare the current ECG to the immediate post-operative baseline — not to the pre-operative ECG and not to a 'normal' ECG. The post-op baseline is the reference point. A new regional ST change from the post-op baseline in a patient with declining hemodynamics is a post-operative MI until proven otherwise. The same ST change that is present and unchanged since admission is part of the expected post-op baseline. The comparison is what makes the interpretation, not the finding itself.

KEY POINTS — CHAPTER 6

Expected vs Dangerous Post-Op ECG Findings

- Expected: sinus tachycardia (treat the cause), nonspecific ST-T changes (monitor), low voltage (monitor for tamponade), first-degree AV block (monitor), new RBBB (monitor). None require emergency intervention in isolation in a hemodynamically stable patient.
- Dangerous: NEW regional ST elevation with reciprocal changes (post-op MI), worsening low voltage + JVD + hemodynamic compromise (tamponade), complete AV block without adequate escape rhythm (pacemaker dependency), new persistent LBBB (echocardiogram, future Sgarbossa requirement).

Post-Op AF and Conduction Changes

- Post-op AF peaks on day 2 — correct electrolytes first (K^+ ≥4.0, Mg^{2+} ≥2.0), then rate control (metoprolol or diltiazem). Cardioversion for hemodynamically unstable AF.
- New LBBB after AVR: Sgarbossa criteria required for all future ischemia evaluation. New complete AV block: use epicardial pacing wires as bridge; permanent pacemaker if persistent > 5-7 days.

Postpericardiotomy Syndrome and Epicardial Wires

- Postpericardiotomy syndrome: 2-6 weeks post-op, diffuse concave ST elevation + PR depression + fever + pleuritic pain. Treat with NSAIDs + colchicine. Do not confuse with STEMI.
- Epicardial wire removal: monitor for tamponade for 4-6 hours after removal. Bedside echo immediately if new hypotension, JVD, or hemodynamic change occurs after wire removal.

REMEMBER THIS

✓ The post-cardiac surgery ECG requires comparison to the immediate post-operative baseline — not to the pre-operative ECG. Expected post-op changes (nonspecific ST-T changes, low voltage, new RBBB, first-degree AV block) are present from the first post-op ECG. What matters is whether a new finding has appeared or a prior finding has worsened. The comparison is the interpretation.

✓ Post-operative AF: correct K^+ and Mg^{2+} before starting antiarrhythmics. Electrolyte correction alone restores sinus rhythm in a significant proportion of post-op AF cases. A patient cardioverted without electrolyte correction will frequently revert. Target K^+ ≥4.0 mEq/L and Mg^{2+} ≥2.0 mEq/L as the first intervention for new post-op AF.

✓ Epicardial wire removal carries a real tamponade risk. Monitor the patient for 4-6 hours post-removal. Any new hemodynamic instability, JVD, or hemodynamic change after removal requires immediate bedside echocardiography to exclude pericardial bleeding and tamponade. This is one of the most commonly missed post-cardiac surgery complications because the clinical team's attention has moved to the next phase of recovery.

Metabolic & Drug-Induced ECG Changes in the ICU

Electrolytes, sedatives, and the QT in critical illness

ICU NURSING · NCLEX · USMLE

The ICU medication list is the most dangerous QTc-prolonging environment in clinical medicine. A critically ill patient may simultaneously receive an antibiotic, an antipsychotic for delirium, an antiemetic, an antifungal, and a sedative — each of which prolongs the QT interval — while also being hypokalemic, hypomagnesemic, and bradycardic from vasopressors. The additive and synergistic effects of these factors on the QT interval are not additive in a linear way: they are potentiating, meaning the combined risk is higher than the sum of the individual risks.

This chapter covers the ECG changes produced by the metabolic derangements and drug classes most commonly encountered in the ICU, and the nursing response to each. Section 7.1 through 7.4 cover the electrolytes. Sections 7.5 through 7.8 cover the drug-induced changes. Section 7.9 provides the integrated QTc management protocol for clinical use.

7.1 Hyperkalemia — Progressive ECG Stages

Hyperkalemia is the electrolyte abnormality with the most predictable and clinically important ECG progression. Recognizing each stage allows the ICU nurse to escalate treatment before the patient reaches the most dangerous stages — wide QRS and sine-wave pattern — where the risk of VF and cardiac arrest is highest.

Stage	K^+ Level	ECG Finding	Immediate Action

1 — Early	**5.5–6.5 mEq/L**	Peaked, narrow, symmetric ('tent-shaped') T waves. Normal PR, normal QRS width. Most prominent in precordial leads V2-V5.	Dietary restriction. Kayexalate or patiromer. Review K^+-retaining medications (ACE inhibitors, ARBs, spironolactone). Recheck K^+ in 4-6 hours.
2 — Moderate	**6.5–7.5 mEq/L**	PR interval prolongation. QRS widening begins (> 0.11 s). P wave amplitude decreases and P waves may become difficult to identify. Peaked T waves persist.	IV calcium gluconate 1 g over 10 min (membrane stabilization). IV insulin 10 units + D50W 25 g (intracellular shift). IV sodium bicarbonate if acidosis present. IV albuterol nebulized.
3 — Severe	**7.5–9.0 mEq/L**	Further QRS widening. P waves absent (atrial paralysis). The QRS-T complex begins to merge, producing the classic sine-wave pattern.	All above agents immediately. Emergency hemodialysis preparation. Continuous cardiac monitoring. Defibrillator at bedside — VF risk is extreme.

4 — Pre-terminal	**> 9.0 mEq/L**	True sine-wave: QRS and T wave are indistinguishable, producing a smooth sinusoidal waveform. Cardiac arrest is imminent.	Emergency hemodialysis if any cardiac output present. Prepare for cardiac arrest (VF). Calcium gluconate IV bolus (repeat dosing). ECMO consultation if available.

HYPERKALEMIA EMERGENCY TREATMENT SEQUENCE — GIVE IN THIS ORDER:

1. IV Calcium gluconate 1 g (10 mL of 10% solution) over 2-5 minutes — membrane stabilization, works within 1-3 minutes. Does NOT lower K^+ — it protects the myocardium while the K^+-lowering agents take effect. Use central line or large peripheral IV (extravasation causes tissue necrosis).

2. IV Regular insulin 10 units + IV Dextrose 50% 25 g (one ampule D50W) simultaneously — shifts K^+ into cells within 20-30 minutes. Recheck glucose at 1 hour (hypoglycemia risk).

3. IV Sodium bicarbonate 50 mEq — shifts K^+ intracellularly via alkalinization. Most effective when metabolic acidosis is present. Less effective at normal pH.

4. Nebulized albuterol 10-20 mg — shifts K^+ intracellularly via beta-2 receptor stimulation. Additive to insulin effect. May cause tachycardia.

5. Emergency hemodialysis — the only treatment that actually REMOVES K^+ from the body. All other agents provide temporary intracellular shifts. Arrange immediately; it is definitive treatment.

6. Recheck K^+ and ECG at 1-2 hours. Repeat calcium gluconate every 30-60 minutes if QRS remains wide.

7.2 Hypokalemia — U Waves and QT Risk

Hypokalemia is the most common electrolyte abnormality in the ICU, driven by diuretic therapy, nasogastric suction, vomiting, and diarrhea. Its ECG effects are less dramatic than hyperkalemia but clinically important: the QTU prolongation it produces significantly increases the risk of torsades de pointes, particularly when combined with QT-prolonging medications.

- ECG findings: flat or inverted T waves, prominent U waves (positive deflections after the T wave, most visible in V2-V4), and apparent QT prolongation (which is actually QTU prolongation when the U wave is incorporated into the measurement).
- Torsades risk: hypokalemia combined with any QT-prolonging medication (antibiotic, antipsychotic, antiemetic, antiarrhythmic) produces a dramatically higher torsades risk than either factor alone. This additive-to-synergistic risk is the primary reason K^+ must be maintained ≥4.0 mEq/L in any ICU patient on QT-prolonging drugs.
- Refractory hypokalemia: if K^+ is not responding to aggressive replacement, check Mg^{2+}. Hypomagnesemia prevents K^+ retention by impairing the Na-K ATPase pump. Replace Mg^{2+} first (target ≥2.0 mEq/L), then K^+ will replete effectively.
- ICU replacement strategy: IV KCl 20-40 mEq over 2-4 hours via central line for K^+ < 3.0 mEq/L or for K^+ 3.0-3.5 mEq/L with symptomatic arrhythmia. Oral KCl for stable K^+ 3.0-3.5 mEq/L in a patient tolerating oral medications. Recheck after each replacement dose.

7.3 Hypomagnesemia — The Silent QT Prolonger

Hypomagnesemia produces minimal distinctive ECG changes of its own, yet it is one of the most clinically important electrolyte abnormalities in the ICU because of its role in amplifying every other QT-prolonging factor. It is common (occurring in 20-60% of ICU patients), frequently undetected (serum magnesium does not reliably reflect intracellular magnesium stores), and almost always coexists with hypokalemia in patients receiving loop diuretics.

Scenario	Clinical Relevance and Action
Hypomagnesemia + QT-prolonging drug	Magnesium deficiency impairs the IKr potassium channel that is blocked by QT-prolonging drugs, making the QT effect of those drugs more pronounced. Any patient receiving a QTc-prolonging ICU medication should have Mg^{2+} checked and repleted to ≥2.0 mEq/L before the drug is started and maintained throughout treatment.

Hypomagnesemia + hypokalemia (most common ICU combination)	Cannot correct K^+ without first correcting Mg^{2+}. Na-K ATPase requires magnesium as a cofactor. Replace IV $MgSO_4$ 2-4 g over 1-2 hours, then resume K^+ replacement and recheck both electrolytes.
Torsades de pointes (regardless of serum Mg^{2+} level)	IV $MgSO_4$ 2 g over 5-15 minutes is first-line treatment for torsades regardless of the measured serum magnesium level. Even a 'normal' serum Mg^{2+} does not reflect intracellular stores adequately. Magnesium stabilizes the IKr channel and shortens the QT interval acutely.
Post-bypass hypomagnesemia	CPB dilutes and wastes magnesium. All post-cardiac surgery patients should have Mg^{2+} checked and repleted to ≥2.0 mEq/L as a routine electrolyte management target, independent of whether arrhythmias are present.

7.4 Hypocalcemia After Massive Transfusion

Hypocalcemia in the ICU occurs in two main contexts: massive transfusion (citrate in blood products chelates ionized calcium, reducing ionized Ca^{2+} acutely) and sepsis-related calcium redistribution. Its ECG effect is QT prolongation from prolonged repolarization — the reverse of hypercalcemia's QT shortening.

- ECG finding: QT prolongation, specifically from lengthening of the ST segment (the interval between the end of the QRS and the beginning of the T wave). The T wave itself is usually normal. This ST segment elongation is distinctive from other causes of QT prolongation where the T wave morphology is more altered.
- Clinical threshold: ionized Ca^{2+} < 1.0 mmol/L is the standard intervention threshold in ICU patients. Total calcium is unreliable in critically ill patients with hypoalbuminemia (calcium is albumin-bound) — always measure ionized calcium in the ICU.
- Massive transfusion protocol: give IV calcium gluconate 1 g for every 4 units of packed red blood cells, FFP, or platelets administered during a massive transfusion. This is a

prophylactic replacement strategy to prevent the progressive ionized calcium decline from citrate chelation.

- Severe hypocalcemia: ionized Ca^{2+} < 0.8 mmol/L can produce cardiac contractility depression, hypotension, laryngospasm, and tetany in addition to QT prolongation. IV calcium gluconate 1-2 g over 10-20 minutes, with continuous ECG monitoring during infusion.

7.5 Propofol Infusion Syndrome ECG

Propofol infusion syndrome (PRIS) is a rare but potentially fatal complication of high-dose, prolonged propofol infusion (typically > 4 mg/kg/h for > 48 hours, though it can occur at lower doses). The ECG finding that should immediately trigger clinical suspicion is one of the most specific drug-induced ECG patterns in the ICU: a new Brugada-like pattern in a sedated patient.

PRIS Feature	Details
ECG pattern	New coved ST elevation in V1-V2 (Type 1 Brugada morphology: steep downsloping ST segment with T wave inversion) appearing in a sedated ICU patient on propofol infusion. The mechanism: propofol blocks cardiac sodium channels (SCN5A) in a manner identical to the loss-of-function mutation causing congenital Brugada syndrome.
Additional ECG findings	Right bundle branch block (new), PR prolongation, wide QRS, and rarely complete AV block in severe cases.
Associated clinical features	Metabolic acidosis (anion gap), rhabdomyolysis (elevated CK, myoglobinuria), renal failure, hyperkalemia, hepatomegaly, and lipemic plasma. The full PRIS picture includes all of these, but the ECG change may be the first detectable sign.

Immediate action	STOP propofol immediately. Switch to an alternative sedation agent (midazolam, dexmedetomidine, ketamine). Notify physician. Obtain CK, lactate, metabolic panel, and urinalysis (myoglobinuria). Continuous ECG monitoring. If Brugada pattern is present with VT/VF: defibrillation per standard protocol. IV lipid emulsion therapy (Intralipid 20%, 1.5 mL/kg bolus) has been used in severe PRIS with some reported benefit.

WHO IS AT HIGHEST RISK FOR PRIS: Children (pediatric ICU patients are at higher risk than adults), patients receiving > 4 mg/kg/h for > 48 hours, patients with high catecholamine states (septic shock, traumatic brain injury), and patients with mitochondrial disorders or carnitine deficiency. Monitoring: obtain a 12-lead ECG and check CK every 24-48 hours in any patient on propofol > 48 hours at doses ≥4 mg/kg/h.

7.6 Sepsis-Associated ECG Changes

Sepsis produces ECG changes through several mechanisms: direct myocardial depression from cytokines (septic cardiomyopathy), demand ischemia from tachycardia and hypotension, electrolyte derangements, and the pro-arrhythmic effects of vasopressor therapy. The ECG in sepsis is neither normal nor diagnostic — it reflects the severity of the physiological insult.

- Sinus tachycardia: the most universal sepsis ECG finding, driven by fever, volume depletion, catecholamine release, and anemia. The rate correlates roughly with severity. Sinus tachycardia in sepsis should not be treated with rate-controlling agents — treat the sepsis.
- Atrial fibrillation: new AF occurs in 5-15% of septic patients. The mechanism is a combination of atrial stretch from fluid resuscitation, autonomic dysregulation, hypoxia, and inflammatory mediator effects on atrial electrophysiology. New AF in sepsis significantly increases ICU mortality and stroke risk.

- Dynamic ST changes (septic cardiomyopathy): diffuse ST depression or T wave inversion can reflect global subendocardial ischemia from reduced coronary perfusion pressure combined with the increased myocardial oxygen demand of sepsis. Troponin is frequently elevated in sepsis from demand ischemia even without obstructive coronary disease.
- QTc prolongation: sepsis itself prolongs the QTc through autonomic dysfunction and electrolyte derangements, and the drugs used to treat sepsis (antibiotics, vasopressors, antifungals) add further QTc risk. QTc monitoring every 12-24 hours is appropriate for any septic ICU patient on QTc-prolonging antibiotics.
- Vasopressor ECG effects: norepinephrine increases HR and may produce demand ischemia at high doses. Epinephrine produces more significant tachycardia and is more arrhythmogenic. Vasopressin has minimal direct cardiac ECG effects but can cause reflex bradycardia at high doses.

7.7 Hypoxia and ECG

Severe hypoxia (SpO_2 < 80%, PaO_2 < 40 mmHg) produces myocardial demand ischemia through a straightforward mechanism: the oxygen supply-demand mismatch causes subendocardial ischemia, which produces the same ECG changes as coronary ischemia. The ECG changes of severe hypoxia are not specific to their cause — they cannot be distinguished from coronary ischemia on the ECG alone.

- ST depression: diffuse or regional ST depression from global subendocardial ischemia. Most visible in leads with tall R waves (I, aVL, V4-V6). The pattern can resemble the left main / diffuse subendocardial pattern (aVR elevation + diffuse depression) if hypoxia is severe enough.
- Sinus tachycardia: compensatory response to the reduced oxygen delivery. HR elevation increases cardiac output but also increases myocardial oxygen demand, worsening the ischemia.
- Atrial arrhythmias: hypoxia is a potent trigger for AF and atrial flutter. New AF in an ICU patient should always prompt a SpO_2 check as part of the immediate assessment.
- Bradycardia and AV block: profound hypoxia (near-fatal levels, PaO_2 < 20 mmHg) can produce vagally-mediated bradycardia

and AV block as the myocardium approaches complete ischemic failure. This is a pre-arrest finding requiring emergency airway management above all else.

- Clinical principle: always correct the hypoxia before interpreting the ECG. An ECG obtained during acute hypoxia reflects the hypoxic insult, not a fixed coronary anatomy. Repeat the ECG after oxygenation is restored — many hypoxia-related ST changes resolve completely with correction of the SpO_2.

7.8 Digoxin in the ICU

Digoxin is used in the ICU primarily for rate control in patients with AF and reduced LVEF who have failed or cannot tolerate other rate-controlling agents. Its narrow therapeutic window, renal clearance dependence, and the potentiating effect of hypokalemia on its toxicity make it one of the highest-risk medications in any critically ill patient.

Finding	Clinical Interpretation and Action
Digoxin EFFECT (therapeutic levels)	Scooped ('Salvador Dali mustache') ST depression in leads with tall R waves (V4-V6, I). This is expected at therapeutic digoxin levels and is NOT evidence of ischemia. Do not order a troponin or a stress test for digoxin-effect ST scooping in an otherwise stable patient.
Digoxin TOXICITY — NPJT with AV block	Non-paroxysmal junctional tachycardia (NPJT): regular narrow-complex tachycardia at 60-120 bpm with retrograde P waves, in a patient with underlying AF — the AF appears 'regularized' because complete AV block is allowing only the junctional escape to conduct. This is the most classic and specific digoxin toxicity arrhythmia.
Digoxin TOXICITY — accelerated junctional rhythm	Regular narrow-complex rhythm at 60-80 bpm in a patient whose underlying rhythm is AF or sinus. The AV junction has enhanced automaticity from digoxin toxicity.
Digoxin TOXICITY — complete AV block	Complete AV block with junctional escape in a patient on digoxin. Hold digoxin, replete K^+ aggressively, consider Digibind.

Digoxin TOXICITY — VT/VF	Life-threatening. Bidirectional VT (alternating QRS axis every other beat) is specifically associated with digoxin toxicity and severe hypokalemia. Defibrillation for VF. NEVER cardiovert digoxin-toxic rhythms — the toxic myocardium has extremely low VF threshold; cardioversion can trigger VF.

DIGOXIN TOXICITY MANAGEMENT IN THE ICU:

1. Hold digoxin immediately. Obtain a stat digoxin level (results typically available in 1-2 hours, but do not wait for results to act if clinical toxicity is clear).

2. Replete K^+ aggressively: target $K^+ \geq 4.0$ mEq/L. Hypokalemia is the most potent potentiator of digoxin toxicity. Repleting K^+ alone may control the arrhythmia if levels are only mildly supra-therapeutic.

3. Digoxin immune Fab (Digibind/DigiFab): administer when hemodynamically significant toxicity is present (VT, complete AV block, hemodynamic compromise). Dosing: (serum digoxin level in ng/mL × weight in kg) ÷ 100 = number of vials. Round up to the nearest whole vial.

4. NEVER cardiovert digoxin-toxic rhythms (except for VF — which requires unsynchronized defibrillation regardless of digoxin status). The toxic myocardium has a dramatically lowered VF threshold; cardioversion energy can trigger VF.

5. Continuous cardiac monitoring. Place defibrillator pads on all patients with digoxin toxicity arrhythmias. The rhythm can deteriorate to VF without warning.

7.9 The ICU QTc Management Protocol

The following protocol integrates QTc monitoring, risk stratification, and drug management into a single clinical workflow for ICU patients. It is designed to be applied at admission and updated daily for any patient receiving one or more QTc-prolonging medications.

ICU QTc MANAGEMENT PROTOCOL — APPLY AT ADMISSION AND UPDATE DAILY:

1. Obtain a 12-lead ECG on admission. Calculate QTc using the Bazett formula: $QTc = QT \div \sqrt{RR}$ (in seconds). Document baseline QTc in the chart.

2. Review the medication list for QTc-prolonging agents: antibiotics (azithromycin, ciprofloxacin, fluconazole), antipsychotics (haloperidol, quetiapine), antiemetics (ondansetron, promethazine), antiarrhythmics (amiodarone, sotalol), methadone, antifungals (voriconazole). Flag any QTc-prolonging agent and document the indication.

3. Check and correct electrolytes: K^+ to ≥4.0 mEq/L, Mg^{2+} to ≥2.0 mEq/L. These are the most modifiable QTc risk factors and should be maintained as targets throughout the ICU stay.

4. Risk stratify: baseline QTc < 0.44 s + single QTc drug + corrected electrolytes = lower risk, monitor daily. QTc 0.44-0.50 s OR multiple QTc drugs = moderate risk, obtain ECG every 12-24 hours, notify provider. QTc > 0.50 s = high risk, notify provider immediately, consider drug substitution, defibrillator at bedside.

5. Daily QTc check: obtain a repeat ECG or use automated QTc measurement from telemetry every 12-24 hours for any patient on QTc-prolonging therapy. Document the value and comparison to baseline.

6. If torsades occurs: IV $MgSO_4$ 2 g over 5-15 minutes (first-line regardless of serum Mg^{2+} level), hold ALL QTc-prolonging medications, correct electrolytes, overdrive pacing at 90-100 bpm if recurrent, do NOT give amiodarone.

AMIODARONE AND TORSADES: Amiodarone is one of the most QTc-prolonging drugs in clinical use — it routinely produces QTc prolongation of 40-60 ms. However, it is paradoxically a very low-risk drug for torsades because it blocks multiple ion channels simultaneously (not just IKr), preventing the transmural dispersion of refractoriness that generates the torsadogenic substrate. This makes amiodarone the EXCEPTION to the 'QTc-prolonging drug = torsades risk' rule. However, amiodarone must still never be given TO TREAT torsades — the mechanism is different from preventing it.

BEDSIDE PEARL The ICU QTc trap: the nurse who checks the QTc today and documents 0.46 s has done the right thing. The nurse who checks the QTc today, sees it is unchanged from yesterday's 0.46 s, and moves on without asking 'what new QTc-prolonging medication was added last night?' has missed the clinical question. QTc monitoring is not about the absolute value in isolation — it is about the trend, the medication changes driving the trend, and the electrolyte status that amplifies every drug effect. Ask three questions every time: What is it today? What was it yesterday? What changed between those two values?

KEY POINTS — CHAPTER 7

Hyperkalemia and Hypokalemia

- Hyperkalemia progression: peaked T waves → PR prolongation + QRS widening → P wave loss + sine wave. At each stage: calcium gluconate first (membrane stabilization, immediate), then insulin + glucose (intracellular shift), then dialysis (removal).
- Hypokalemia: flat T waves + U waves + QTU prolongation. Target K^+ ≥4.0 mEq/L in all ICU patients on QTc-prolonging drugs. Cannot correct K^+ without first correcting Mg^{2+}.

Propofol Infusion Syndrome and Digoxin

- PRIS: new Brugada-like coved ST elevation in V1-V2 in a sedated patient on propofol > 48 hours at high doses. Stop propofol immediately, switch sedation agent, obtain CK and lactate.
- Digoxin toxicity: NPJT + regularized AF is pathognomonic. NEVER cardiovert. Hold digoxin, replete K^+, Digibind for hemodynamically significant toxicity. Bidirectional VT = severe toxicity.

QTc Management

- QTc > 0.50 s: notify provider immediately, review all QTc-prolonging drugs, correct K^+ and Mg^{2+}, defibrillator at bedside. Torsades treatment: IV $MgSO_4$ 2 g first-line, hold all QTc drugs, overdrive pacing if recurrent. Never give amiodarone FOR torsades (it is safe to use amiodarone in other contexts despite QTc prolongation).

- Ask three questions daily for every patient on QTc-prolonging therapy: What is the QTc today? What was it yesterday? What changed between those values?

REMEMBER THIS

✓ Calcium gluconate is the first agent in hyperkalemia because it works in minutes and buys time for the K^+-lowering agents to act. It does not lower the K^+ level — it stabilizes the myocardial membrane against the depolarizing effect of high extracellular K^+. Give it first, then give insulin + glucose to shift K^+ intracellularly, then arrange dialysis to remove it. The sequence matters: membrane stabilization → intracellular shift → removal.

✓ Cannot correct hypokalemia without correcting hypomagnesemia. This is the most commonly missed two-part replacement principle in the ICU. If K^+ is not rising despite aggressive replacement, check Mg^{2+} and replete it first. The Na-K ATPase pump that retains intracellular potassium requires magnesium as a cofactor — without adequate Mg^{2+}, K^+ is continuously lost renally regardless of how much is given.

✓ The ICU QTc protocol requires three concurrent actions, not one: check the QTc value, review every medication for QTc risk, and verify the electrolyte targets (K^+ ≥4.0, Mg^{2+} ≥2.0). A QTc of 0.49 s with K^+ 2.8 and Mg^{2+} 1.4 on haloperidol + azithromycin + ondansetron simultaneously is a patient in danger. The same QTc of 0.49 s with normal electrolytes on a single agent is a patient who needs monitoring. The number alone does not tell the story.

Hemodynamics and the ECG

When the ECG explains why the numbers are wrong

ICU NURSING · RAPID RESPONSE · USMLE

A patient's blood pressure drops. The cardiac output falls. The central venous pressure rises. These hemodynamic numbers tell you that something is wrong. The ECG is the tool that most reliably explains why — whether it is a rhythm problem reducing stroke volume, a pericardial process preventing ventricular filling, an ischemic event reducing contractility, or a right heart failure changing the physiology of the entire circulatory system.

This chapter bridges the two parallel data streams that every ICU nurse manages simultaneously: the hemodynamic numbers from the monitor and invasive lines, and the ECG from the cardiac monitor. The skill is reading both together, recognizing when they explain each other, and identifying the specific ECG finding that dictates the next hemodynamic intervention.

8.1 The ECG-Hemodynamic Framework

When hemodynamic numbers are abnormal, the ECG should always be examined as a first-line diagnostic tool. Five ECG-hemodynamic pairings account for the majority of cases where the ECG explains the hemodynamic picture:

Hemodynamic Picture	ECG Finding That Explains It	Primary Diagnosis
Hypotension + reduced CO + pulmonary edema	Regional ST elevation (anterior, lateral, or inferior) with or without reciprocal changes	Cardiogenic shock from acute MI
Hypotension + elevated CVP/JVD + muffled sounds	Low voltage + electrical alternans + sinus tachycardia	Cardiac tamponade

Hypotension + elevated CVP + clear lungs (no pulmonary edema)	Inferior ST elevation (II/III/aVF) + V4R positive	RV infarction (preload-dependent failure)
Hypotension + elevated pulmonary pressures + right heart strain signs	New S1Q3T3 + new RBBB + sinus tachycardia (new vs prior ECG)	Massive pulmonary embolism
Unexplained hypotension in a monitored patient with an organized rhythm	Organized ECG rhythm + no pulse confirmed on palpation	PEA — search H's and T's immediately

8.2 Cardiogenic Shock — Two ECG Patterns, Two Anatomies

Cardiogenic shock is defined by sustained hypotension (SBP < 90 mmHg) with evidence of organ hypoperfusion despite adequate preload, caused by primary cardiac dysfunction. The ECG in cardiogenic shock serves two functions: it identifies the likely cause (regional vs global ischemia), and it determines the urgency and direction of coronary intervention.

Pattern 1 — Regional STEMI with Cardiogenic Shock

- ECG: regional ST elevation confined to a specific territory (anterior V1-V5, inferior II/III/aVF, or lateral I/aVL/V5-V6) with reciprocal ST depression in mirror-image leads.
- Mechanism: occlusion of a single major coronary artery producing regional LV dysfunction sufficient to impair global cardiac output. The most common cause: large anterior STEMI from proximal LAD occlusion (the 'widow-maker' territory — the largest single LV territory from any coronary artery).
- Hemodynamic profile: reduced CO, elevated PCWP (pulmonary edema from LV failure), reduced SVR from catecholamine vasodilation, hypotension. Troponin will be dramatically elevated.
- Action: emergent PCI without delay. Every minute of ongoing LAD occlusion in cardiogenic shock adds irreversible

myocardial damage. Mechanical circulatory support (IABP, Impella, or VA-ECMO) may be placed before or during PCI for highest-risk patients.

Pattern 2 — Diffuse Subendocardial Ischemia (Left Main / Multivessel)

- ECG: diffuse ST depression in ≥6 leads (V2-V6, I, II, aVL) with ST elevation ONLY in lead aVR and sometimes V1. No regional ST elevation in any standard STEMI territory.
- Mechanism: critical left main or severe triple-vessel disease producing global subendocardial ischemia. The entire LV is underperfused simultaneously. This produces a hemodynamic picture that is often worse than regional STEMI because no myocardial territory is spared.
- Hemodynamic profile: similar to regional STEMI shock but often more severe, as the entire LV is affected. Troponin elevation, reduced CO, pulmonary edema, hypotension.
- Action: emergent angiography — the ECG pattern identifies the most hostile coronary anatomy. Mechanical circulatory support is more frequently required upfront. CABG may be preferred over PCI for left main disease depending on anatomy.

THE KEY DISTINCTION BETWEEN THE TWO PATTERNS: Regional STEMI shock shows ST ELEVATION in a specific territory. Left main/multivessel shock shows ST DEPRESSION everywhere with aVR elevation — no regional elevation. This distinction matters because the absence of regional ST elevation in the diffuse depression pattern frequently delays cath lab activation; the team waits for troponin confirmation instead of recognizing the ECG pattern as itself indicating emergent intervention. The aVR elevation + diffuse depression pattern demands the same urgency as a classic STEMI.

8.3 RV Failure on the ECG

Right ventricular failure in the ICU produces a hemodynamic pattern that is the opposite of LV failure: elevated right-sided pressures with a relatively clear left heart, producing JVD without pulmonary edema (unless biventricular failure supervenes). The ECG provides specific clues to both the presence and the severity of RV strain.

ECG Finding	Clinical Significance in RV Failure
Right axis deviation (axis > +90°)	The dominant electrical vector has shifted rightward, reflecting RV hypertrophy or acute RV pressure overload. New right axis deviation in an ICU patient with hemodynamic deterioration should prompt immediate evaluation for acute RV strain (PE, ARDS-related pulmonary hypertension, acute RV infarction).
S1Q3T3 pattern	S wave in lead I + Q wave in lead III + T wave inversion in lead III. Sensitivity for PE is approximately 20% — present in about 1 in 5 confirmed PE cases. Specificity is higher when all three components are present simultaneously and represent a NEW finding compared to a prior ECG.
New RBBB	The right bundle branch is sensitive to acute RV pressure elevation — it can become functionally blocked from ischemia or mechanical compression when RV pressure rises acutely. New RBBB in the context of hemodynamic instability and elevated right-sided pressures is a marker of severe acute RV strain.
T wave inversion V1-V3 (RV strain pattern)	The RV-facing precordial leads show T wave inversion reflecting abnormal RV repolarization from pressure overload or ischemia. This pattern is identical in appearance to Wellens-type T wave inversion (anterior LAD territory) — always compare to a prior ECG to determine whether the finding is new (acute RV strain or Wellens) vs stable (chronic cor pulmonale from COPD or pulmonary hypertension).
P pulmonale (peaked P waves ≥ 2.5 mm in II)	Right atrial enlargement from chronically elevated RV pressure. This finding on a serial ICU ECG in a patient with new hemodynamic deterioration suggests acute-on-chronic RV failure from a new insult superimposed on a pre-existing pulmonary hypertension substrate.

RV FAILURE HEMODYNAMIC TRIAD: JVD (elevated right heart pressure) + hypotension (reduced CO from RV failure) + clear lungs or minimal pulmonary edema (the LV is underfilled, not overloaded). This pattern is the opposite of LV failure (pulmonary edema + clear neck veins from compensated right heart). Recognizing the RV failure pattern on clinical exam and correlating it with the ECG right-heart-strain signs guides the correct hemodynamic intervention: volume expansion to maintain RV preload (not diuresis), vasopressors to maintain RV perfusion pressure, and treat the underlying cause (PE, acute cor pulmonale, RV infarction).

8.4 Pericardial Effusion and Hemodynamic Compromise

A pericardial effusion becomes hemodynamically significant when its volume and the rate of accumulation produce enough intrapericardial pressure to impair ventricular diastolic filling. The ECG cannot diagnose an effusion — that requires echocardiography — but it can raise the clinical suspicion that leads to the echo before the patient decompensates.

ECG Findings Suggesting Significant Pericardial Effusion

- Low voltage: QRS amplitude < 5 mm in all limb leads. Reflects the electrical insulating effect of the surrounding pericardial fluid. Low voltage alone is not diagnostic of tamponade — it indicates the presence of fluid without quantifying hemodynamic significance.
- Electrical alternans: beat-to-beat alternation in QRS amplitude, reflecting the heart swinging within the fluid-filled pericardial sac. When present with low voltage and hemodynamic compromise, electrical alternans has high specificity for tamponade. When present without hemodynamic compromise, it indicates a large effusion that requires echocardiographic monitoring and likely drainage.
- Sinus tachycardia: compensatory mechanism from reduced stroke volume. In tamponade, tachycardia is often the first measurable sign of hemodynamic compromise, appearing before hypotension.
- Pericarditis ECG pattern (Stage 1): diffuse concave ST elevation with PR depression may be present if the effusion is

inflammatory in origin. Post-cardiac surgery, post-MI (Dressler syndrome), viral pericarditis, and malignant pericardial disease can all produce inflammatory effusions with the concurrent Stage 1 pericarditis pattern.

TAMPONADE CLINICAL ASSESSMENT PROTOCOL:

1. Assess hemodynamics: HR, BP, pulse pressure (narrowing pulse pressure is an early sign — systolic falls, diastolic rises as the pericardial pressure restricts stroke volume).

2. Assess for JVD: elevated jugular venous pressure from impaired RV filling. Kussmaul's sign (paradoxical rise in JVP with inspiration) suggests constrictive physiology but is less reliable than in constrictive pericarditis.

3. Auscultate heart sounds: muffled or distant heart sounds reflect the acoustic damping effect of surrounding fluid. Beck's triad: hypotension + JVD + muffled sounds.

4. Measure pulsus paradoxus: exaggerated fall in systolic BP (≥ 10 mmHg) during normal inspiration. Have the patient breathe normally; measure systolic BP at end-expiration and at peak inspiration. A ≥ 10 mmHg fall confirms significant tamponade physiology.

5. Bedside echocardiography immediately if any two of the above signs are present: RV and/or RA collapse during diastole on echo = tamponade confirmed. Pericardiocentesis preparation.

8.5 Pulmonary Hypertension — Chronic vs Acute Decompensation

Patients with chronic pulmonary hypertension (from COPD, idiopathic pulmonary arterial hypertension, or connective tissue disease) are a unique ICU subpopulation because their baseline ECG already shows RVH changes. When these patients deteriorate hemodynamically, the ECG challenge is distinguishing a new acute insult from worsening of their chronic baseline.

ECG Comparison	Clinical Significance

Chronic stable RVH on serial ECGs (stable right axis, stable R > S in V1, stable T inversions V1-V3)	This is the expected baseline for a patient with established chronic pulmonary hypertension. Hemodynamic deterioration in this patient should trigger a search for a superimposed acute process (infection, PE on top of pulmonary hypertension, arrhythmia) rather than attributing the deterioration to the chronic ECG pattern.
NEW worsening of RVH pattern vs prior (new or worsening right axis deviation, new or worsening T inversions V1-V3, new S1Q3T3 or new RBBB)	An acute change from the patient's established chronic baseline indicates a new acute RV insult. In a pulmonary hypertension patient, differential: acute PE (most important to exclude), acute pneumonia causing further hypoxia and pulmonary vasoconstriction, or intrinsic worsening of pulmonary vascular disease.
Loss of P pulmonale that was previously present (P waves become less peaked or narrower)	This counter-intuitive finding can indicate improvement in right atrial pressure (if the underlying cause is treated) OR it can indicate loss of atrial activity from severe AF or a rhythm change. Correlate with clinical trajectory and rhythm strip.

> **THE PRIOR ECG IS THE MOST VALUABLE TOOL:** In any patient with known chronic pulmonary disease, the prior ECG determines what is baseline. A T wave inversion in V1-V3 that has been present and unchanged on 8 serial ECGs is chronic cor pulmonale; the same finding appearing for the first time on today's ECG is acute RV strain until proven otherwise. Always obtain prior ECGs before concluding that right heart strain findings are chronic.

8.6 Vasopressor Effects on the ECG

Vasopressors are among the most commonly administered medications in the ICU. Each agent in the vasopressor class has a distinct receptor profile that produces specific cardiac and ECG effects. Understanding these effects allows the ICU nurse to anticipate ECG changes that are expected from the vasopressor itself versus changes that indicate a new cardiac problem.

Agent	Receptor Profile	Expected ECG Effects

Norepinephrine (first-line vasopressor)	Alpha-1 (dominant) + beta-1 (moderate)	Reflex bradycardia from the alpha-1 mediated rise in BP (baroreceptor reflex). Moderate increases in HR at lower doses. At high doses: demand ischemia from increased myocardial O_2 consumption + reduced diastolic filling time from tachycardia. Monitor for new ST depression or T wave changes at high doses (≥ 0.5 mcg/kg/min).
Epinephrine (anaphylaxis, cardiac arrest, refractory shock)	Alpha-1 + beta-1 + beta-2 (all significant)	Sinus tachycardia (often marked — HR 120-150 bpm at doses > 0.1 mcg/kg/min). High risk of demand ischemia and arrhythmia (PVCs, VT) from potent beta-1 stimulation. Any new VT, sustained PVC burden, or new ST changes during epinephrine infusion should prompt provider notification and dose review.
Vasopressin (adjunct to norepinephrine)	V1 receptors (vascular smooth muscle) — no direct cardiac receptor activity	Reflex bradycardia from the vasopressor effect (similar to norepinephrine's reflex mechanism). Coronary vasoconstriction at high doses can produce demand ischemia. At standard ICU doses (0.03-0.04 units/min), cardiac ECG effects are minimal.

Dopamine (dose-dependent effects)	D1 (low dose) → beta-1 (medium dose) → alpha-1 (high dose)	Beta-1 stimulation at intermediate doses (5-10 mcg/kg/min) produces tachycardia and increased arrhythmia risk. Higher rates of AF and VT than norepinephrine in septic shock (supported by clinical trial data). Generally avoid as first-line vasopressor in tachycardic patients or those with a history of AF.
Phenylephrine (pure alpha-1 agonist)	Alpha-1 only — no direct cardiac receptor activity	Reflex bradycardia (sometimes marked) from pure alpha-1 mediated BP elevation without beta-1 HR support. Can produce significant bradycardia in patients with baseline conduction disease. If HR drops below 50 bpm on phenylephrine: notify provider; consider switching to norepinephrine.

8.7 Volume Status and the ECG

Volume status affects the ECG through its effect on cardiac chamber dimensions, heart rate, and myocardial oxygen demand. While the ECG is not a direct measurement of volume status, several ECG patterns correlate with volume-related hemodynamic states that are clinically actionable.

- Sinus tachycardia from hypovolemia: one of the most common causes of tachycardia in the ICU. HR > 100 bpm that does not have an obvious alternative explanation (fever, pain, anxiety, drug effect) should prompt an assessment of volume status before initiating rate-controlling therapy. Giving a rate-controlling agent to a tachycardic hypovolemic patient removes the compensatory mechanism and can precipitate hemodynamic collapse.

- QRS amplitude changes with volume: severe dehydration and hypovolemia can reduce QRS amplitude (low voltage from reduced ventricular filling and smaller stroke volume). Conversely, volume overload and massive fluid resuscitation can reduce QRS amplitude from dilutional hyponatremia and generalized tissue edema. Neither pattern is specific, but a change in QRS amplitude from admission to 48 hours later in an ICU patient should trigger a volume status reassessment.
- P wave morphology and atrial filling: in severe hypovolemia, P wave amplitude may decrease as right atrial filling pressure falls. In volume overload, broad notched P waves (P mitrale — bifid P wave in leads I and II) can develop from elevated left atrial filling pressure. These are subtle and not primary diagnostic findings, but they form part of the ECG evidence base for volume assessment.
- Volume and arrhythmia: both hypovolemia and volume overload are independent triggers for atrial and ventricular arrhythmias. Hypovolemia causes adrenergic activation that increases myocardial irritability. Volume overload causes atrial and ventricular stretch that promotes ectopy and re-entry. New arrhythmias in an ICU patient should always include volume status in the differential.
- The integrated hemodynamic-ECG assessment: in the ICU, the ECG should never be read in isolation from the hemodynamic data. MAP, CVP, CO, PCWP, and SpO_2 context transforms the meaning of any ECG finding. A sinus tachycardia at 118 bpm means something different in a patient with MAP 55, CVP 2, and a new fever than it does in a patient with MAP 82, CVP 12, and a vasopressor infusion running.

8.8 The Integrated Hemodynamic-ECG Assessment Protocol

The following protocol provides a structured approach for any ICU patient with new hemodynamic deterioration. It uses the ECG as a first-line diagnostic tool to narrow the differential before more invasive or time-consuming investigations are initiated.

HEMODYNAMIC DETERIORATION ECG ASSESSMENT PROTOCOL:

1. Obtain a 12-lead ECG immediately — within 5 minutes of any new hemodynamic deterioration (SBP drop ≥ 20 mmHg from prior baseline, MAP < 65 on vasopressors, new oxygen requirement, or altered mental status of unclear cause).
2. Compare to the most recent prior ECG from this admission — not the pre-admission baseline. The question is: what has CHANGED since the last tracing?
3. Apply the ECG-hemodynamic framework (Section 8.1): does the ECG show regional ST elevation (STEMI/RV infarction), diffuse depression + aVR elevation (left main), low voltage + alternans (tamponade), S1Q3T3 + new RBBB (PE), or organized rhythm without a pulse (PEA)?
4. If the ECG shows a specific pattern matching one of the five ECG-hemodynamic pairings: activate the corresponding response immediately (cath lab, echo, RRT/Code Blue).
5. If the ECG is unchanged from the prior tracing: the ECG is not explaining the hemodynamic deterioration. Pursue non-ECG causes: bleeding, infection, medication effect, equipment failure, or a non-cardiac organ system failure.
6. Document the ECG finding, the comparison to the prior tracing, the clinical assessment, and the action taken. Include the time of ECG acquisition and the time of provider notification with your documentation.

BEDSIDE PEARL The hemodynamic-ECG integration principle: when a patient's blood pressure is falling and you cannot explain why from the clinical picture, obtain a 12-lead ECG before escalating vasopressors. Adding more vasopressor to a patient in tamponade, to a patient with an obstructive RV infarction who needs fluids, or to a patient with a new VT that the monitor is counting as a normal rate because the QRS is wide — each of these is the wrong intervention applied to a problem that the ECG would have identified in 60 seconds. The ECG is the fastest diagnostic tool available in the ICU. Use it first.

KEY POINTS — CHAPTER 8

The Five ECG-Hemodynamic Pairings

- Regional ST elevation + shock = cardiogenic shock from MI — emergent PCI.

- Diffuse ST depression + aVR elevation + shock = left main/multivessel — emergent angiography with same urgency as STEMI.
- Low voltage + electrical alternans + Beck's triad = tamponade — bedside echo immediately, pericardiocentesis.
- S1Q3T3 + new RBBB + sinus tachycardia + hypotension = massive PE — systemic thrombolytics or embolectomy.
- Organized rhythm + no pulse = PEA — CPR + epinephrine + H's and T's.

RV Failure and Volume

- RV failure ECG signs: right axis deviation, S1Q3T3, new RBBB, T inversions V1-V3, P pulmonale. Hemodynamic pattern: JVD + hypotension + clear lungs. Treat with volume (not diuretics), vasopressors for RV perfusion, and fix the underlying cause.
- Sinus tachycardia in the ICU: always find the cause before treating the rate. Tachycardia from hypovolemia is compensatory — rate control in a hypovolemic patient removes the compensation and precipitates collapse.

Vasopressors and ECG

- Norepinephrine: reflex bradycardia expected; demand ischemia risk at high doses. Epinephrine: marked tachycardia + VT risk from beta-1 stimulation. Phenylephrine: marked reflex bradycardia possible. Dopamine: highest AF and VT risk — avoid in tachycardic patients.
- Any new ST changes, new VT, or significant HR change during vasopressor infusion requires provider notification and medication review.

REMEMBER THIS

✓ When hemodynamics are deteriorating, the 12-lead ECG is the first diagnostic tool — faster than a STAT echo, faster than an ABG, faster than a troponin. It answers the most important diagnostic question (is there a cardiac electrical cause for this deterioration?) in under 60 seconds. The five

ECG-hemodynamic pairings cover the most common life-threatening explanations. If the ECG matches one of them, act on it before pursuing any other investigation.

✓ The prior ECG is the reference point, not normal values. In the ICU, many patients have ECG abnormalities at baseline. The question is always: what has changed from the most recent prior tracing? A new right axis deviation, a new low voltage, a new T wave inversion in V1-V3 — each of these is significant because it is new. The same finding that has been stable on serial tracings is a baseline feature, not an acute finding.

✓ Volume status and the ECG are linked in both directions. Sinus tachycardia that appears to need rate control may actually need a fluid bolus. New AF in a patient who has been stable for three days may reflect atrial stretch from volume overload. New VT in a previously stable patient may reflect hypokalemia and hypomagnesemia from aggressive diuresis. The hemodynamic context transforms the meaning of every arrhythmia in the ICU.

Rapid Response — When to Activate and What to Bring

ECG-triggered RRT activation criteria

RAPID RESPONSE · ER NURSING · ACLS

The rapid response team (RRT) exists to prevent cardiac arrest. The evidence base for RRT programs consistently shows that early activation — before a patient deteriorates to the point of pulselessness — reduces in-hospital cardiac arrest rates, ICU transfers, and mortality. The ECG is one of the most reliable early warning tools available for identifying which patients on a general ward are about to deteriorate, but only if the nurse who reads the rhythm knows which findings demand an immediate RRT call.

This chapter provides the ECG-specific activation criteria that should trigger an RRT call, the first 120-second assessment sequence when the RRT arrives, the equipment checklist, and the bedside decision algorithms for the two most common arrhythmia scenarios the RRT encounters: bradycardia and tachycardia.

9.1 ECG-Triggered RRT Activation Criteria

Most RRT activation criteria focus on vital signs: HR, BP, RR, SpO_2, and clinical concern. ECG-specific criteria are less commonly listed but are equally important — because certain rhythm findings on a telemetry monitor predict imminent deterioration even when the vital signs are still in the acceptable range. The following ECG findings should trigger an immediate RRT call regardless of the patient's current blood pressure or clinical appearance.

ECG Finding	Why It Triggers RRT	Do Not Wait For

New Mobitz II AV block (fixed PR, sudden dropped QRS, wide QRS)	Mobitz II can progress to complete AV block and asystole without any warning. In a pacemaker-dependen t patient or a patient without an adequate escape rhythm, this is cardiac arrest waiting to happen.	Symptoms. Asymptomatic Mobitz II is still a Class I pacemaker indication. Activate RRT and TCP preparation before the patient becomes hemodynamically compromised.
New complete AV block with wide ventricular escape (QRS ≥ 0.12 s, rate 20-40 bpm)	Wide escape rhythm at 20-40 bpm is unstable. Atropine will not work (infranodal block has no vagal innervation). Without TCP, this patient has no adequate pacing mechanism.	BP to drop below threshold. Act at rhythm identification. TCP pads should be applied before any other intervention.
Sustained VT (any morphology) > 30 seconds on the monitor	Sustained VT is hemodynamically significant regardless of the momentary BP. It can deteriorate to VF within seconds.	The patient to report symptoms. Some patients remain conscious during VT for 1-2 minutes before losing consciousness.
New wide-complex irregular tachycardia > 200 bpm (pre-excited AF pattern)	VF risk is extreme if AV-nodal blockers are given. The RRT must arrive before any medication is administered so that the correct management (procainamide or defibrillation) can be initiated.	Any nurse or provider to administer adenosine, verapamil, or diltiazem. The RRT call and the medication hold happen simultaneously.

Electrical alternans + low voltage + tachycardia in a non-monitored patient	This ECG triad identifies cardiac tamponade before Beck's triad is fully manifest clinically. Tamponade can deteriorate to PEA cardiac arrest within minutes.	Full clinical signs of tamponade to appear. The ECG pattern alone is sufficient to activate the RRT and prepare for emergency echo and pericardiocentesis.
Any organized rhythm in an unresponsive patient (possible PEA)	If the patient is unresponsive and the monitor shows an organized rhythm, the default is cardiac arrest until a pulse is confirmed. RRT or Code Blue activation, CPR, and pulse check occur simultaneously.	Pulse check to confirm before calling the RRT. Call while checking.

9.2 The First 120 Seconds — Arrive, Assess, Announce, Act

When the RRT arrives at a bedside, the first 120 seconds determine the trajectory of the event. Disorganized arrivals — multiple people talking simultaneously, no clear assessment sequence, equipment not ready — delay the critical interventions. The following sequence establishes rapid situational awareness and assigns the first actions before a physician has arrived.

RRT FIRST 120-SECOND SEQUENCE:

1. ARRIVE: Identify the RRT leader as you enter the room. One voice, one direction. Announce: 'RRT is here. I am [name], I will lead. Everyone else support.' Silence extraneous conversations.

2. ASSESS (0-30 seconds): Simultaneously: (a) Look at the patient — conscious or unresponsive? Breathing? Colour? (b) Look at the monitor — rate, rhythm, QRS width, ST segment status. (c) Look at the numbers — BP, SpO_2, RR. Do not speak yet.

3. ANNOUNCE (30-45 seconds): State the finding clearly to the team: 'Patient is [conscious/unresponsive]. Monitor shows [VT / complete AV block / organized rhythm, no pulse visible]. BP [X], SpO_2 [X].'

4. ACT (45-120 seconds): Based on the announced finding, initiate the first intervention: defibrillator pads applied (VT/VF), TCP pads applied (symptomatic bradycardia), CPR initiated (pulseless), 12-lead ECG obtained (new rhythm, stable patient), SBAR call to physician initiated (stable arrhythmia requiring orders).

5. DELEGATE: Once the first intervention is in progress, assign specific tasks: 'You — obtain IV access. You — prepare atropine/amiodarone/adenosine as appropriate. You — call the physician now with SBAR. You — document with time-stamps from this moment.'

6. REASSESS at 2-minute intervals: rhythm, hemodynamics, and response to intervention. Adjust the plan based on the patient's trajectory.

9.3 What to Bring — The RRT Equipment Checklist

The RRT cart or bag should contain every item needed to manage any rhythm emergency on a general ward before the patient can be transferred to the ICU. The following checklist covers the minimum equipment standard. If any item is missing when the RRT is called, it must be sourced immediately from the nearest nursing station or crash cart.

Category	Items and Notes
Cardiac monitor / defibrillator	Biphasic defibrillator with SYNC capability. Pacing capability (transcutaneous). Pads (anterior-apical and anterior-posterior sets). Rhythm strip paper. Multi-lead capability (at minimum leads I, II, V1). Confirm battery charge and pad integrity before every shift.
Airway and oxygen	BVM with mask (appropriate sizes). Supplemental oxygen (portable tank or wall connection adapter). Suction. Oral airway adjuncts (nasopharyngeal/oropharyngeal airways). Laryngoscope and ETT (for RRT teams with intubation scope).

IV access	Large-bore peripheral IV catheters (≥ 18-gauge). IV tubing. Normal saline 500 mL bags (×2). IV push flush syringes. Tourniquet. If no IV access in 2 attempts: IO drill and IO needles.
Medications — rhythm	Atropine 1 mg/10 mL (×3). Adenosine 6 mg/2 mL (×2). Amiodarone 150 mg/3 mL (×2). Lidocaine 100 mg/5 mL (×2). Procainamide 1 g/10 mL (×1). Magnesium sulfate 2 g/50 mL (×1). Calcium gluconate 1 g/10 mL (×2).
Medications — resuscitation	Epinephrine 1 mg/10 mL (×5). Sodium bicarbonate 50 mEq/50 mL (×2). Dextrose 50% 25 g/50 mL (×2). Naloxone 0.4 mg/mL (×2). Normal saline 0.9% 10 mL flush syringes (×10).
Documentation	Pre-printed RRT documentation form with time-stamp fields. Pen. Cardiac rhythm strip roll (to document each rhythm change during the event). Patient identifier wristband scanner if available.
Communication	Direct line to the physician covering the unit. Cardiology consult number. Cath lab activation number. Transport team number for ICU transfer.

9.4 Bradycardia RRT Algorithm — Wide vs Narrow in 60 Seconds

Bradycardia at an RRT is the most common scenario where the wrong first intervention is given. The decision between atropine and TCP is determined entirely by the QRS width — yet this assessment is frequently skipped in the urgency of the moment, leading to atropine being given to a patient with infranodal complete AV block (where it will have no effect) while TCP is delayed.

Bradycardia Type	First Intervention and Rationale

NARROW QRS bradycardia (QRS < 0.12 s) HR < 50 bpm with hemodynamic compromise	Atropine 0.5 mg IV first-line. Repeat every 3-5 minutes to maximum 3 mg. Narrow QRS confirms the escape or block is at or above the AV node — vagolytic therapy (atropine) increases AV nodal conduction. Expected causes: sinus bradycardia, first-degree AV block with slow sinus rate, Wenckebach (Mobitz I), junctional bradycardia. If atropine works: monitor, treat the underlying cause (inferior MI, drug effect, vagal). If atropine fails: TCP.
WIDE QRS bradycardia (QRS ≥ 0.12 s) HR < 50 bpm with hemodynamic compromise	TCP immediately — do NOT give atropine first. Wide QRS confirms the pacemaker or block is infranodal (below the His bundle). Purkinje fibers and ventricular myocardium have no significant vagal innervation — atropine will have no effect. Giving atropine wastes 3-5 critical minutes while the patient continues at 28 bpm. TCP: apply pads, set rate 70-80 bpm, increase mA until electrical and mechanical capture confirmed. Analgesia and sedation for patient comfort.
Hemodynamically STABLE bradycardia of any QRS width	Assess and notify — no immediate intervention required. Identify the cause: check medications (beta-blockers, digoxin, diltiazem), electrolytes (hyperkalemia), prior cardiac history (conduction disease, inferior MI), Holter strip review for AV block classification. Provider notification with SBAR. Prepare atropine and TCP as standby in case of deterioration.
Bradycardia + chest pain or inferior ST elevation	Obtain right-sided ECG (V4R) immediately before any medication. If inferior STEMI + AV block: Wenckebach is the most likely type (narrow QRS, responds to atropine). Atropine appropriate first-line. RCA reperfusion (PCI) will resolve the AV block. Do NOT give nitrates until V4R is obtained and RV infarction is excluded.

TCP TECHNIQUE AT THE RRT BEDSIDE: Apply pads in anteroapical position (most rapid) or anteroposterior if time permits. Set rate 70-80 bpm. Start at 60 mA and increase in 10 mA increments until electrical capture (a wide paced QRS follows every spike) AND mechanical capture (a palpable pulse with each captured beat — always confirm by palpation, not just the monitor). IV analgesia (fentanyl 25-50 mcg) and IV sedation (midazolam 1-2 mg) as soon as IV access is established — TCP is painful and patient comfort affects compliance with the pacing pads.

9.5 Tachycardia RRT Algorithm — The Four-Branch Decision

Every tachycardia at an RRT falls into one of four branches based on two binary assessments: QRS width (narrow or wide) and hemodynamic stability (stable or unstable). The branch determines the intervention. The assessment takes 30 seconds. The intervention follows immediately.

QRS	Stability	First Intervention
Narrow	**STABLE**	Vagal maneuvers first (Valsalva, carotid sinus massage if no contraindications). If no response: IV adenosine 6 mg rapid push + 20 mL saline flush. If no response: IV adenosine 12 mg. If no response: diltiazem or metoprolol IV for rate control (confirm no WPW before administering).
Narrow	**UNSTABLE**	Synchronized cardioversion immediately: 50-100 J biphasic. SYNC ON, confirm sync markers on QRS peaks. Sedate if time permits (do not delay cardioversion). Most narrow-complex tachycardias with hemodynamic compromise are AF, flutter, or AVNRT — all respond well to synchronized cardioversion.

Wide	**STABLE**	12-lead ECG and Brugada algorithm. Treat as VT unless SVT with aberrancy is confirmed by specific criteria. IV amiodarone 150 mg over 10 minutes. Pads applied, defibrillator on standby. NEVER give verapamil, diltiazem, or adenosine to an unconfirmed wide-complex tachycardia.
Wide	**UNSTABLE**	Synchronized cardioversion immediately: 100 J biphasic. SYNC ON. If polymorphic (varying morphology, may be torsades): UNSYNCHRONIZED 200 J (cannot reliably sync to a changing QRS). If pulseless: CPR + defibrillation 200 J unsynchronized — this is now a cardiac arrest, not a tachycardia RRT.

WIDE + IRREGULAR + > 200 BPM + WPW = PRE-EXCITED AF: This tachycardia does not fit neatly into the four-branch algorithm because the standard narrow-complex treatments (adenosine, verapamil, diltiazem) are absolutely contraindicated. If the patient is stable: IV procainamide. If unstable: unsynchronized defibrillation 200 J. Hold ALL AV-nodal blocking agents. Identify this pattern before any medication is administered.

9.6 RRT SBAR — The Activation Call and the Physician Call

Two SBAR communications occur during most RRT events: the activation call (from the bedside nurse to the RRT) and the physician call (from the RRT leader to the responsible physician for orders and disposition). Both should follow the SBAR structure and should be practiced until they become automatic.

SBAR — RRT ACTIVATION CALL

S: This is [Name], RN on [Unit], Room [X]. I am activating the rapid response team for [patient name], a [age]-year-old [sex].

B: The patient was admitted for [primary diagnosis]. Current vital signs: HR [X], BP [X], SpO_2 [X]%. The telemetry monitor shows [specific rhythm finding: new Mobitz II / complete AV block / VT / pre-excited AF / organized rhythm, no pulse]. This is NEW compared to the prior tracing from [time].

A: I am concerned this patient is at risk for [hemodynamic collapse / cardiac arrest / VF] based on the ECG finding and current clinical status.

R: I am requesting the rapid response team to the bedside immediately. I am holding all rhythm-active medications pending RRT assessment. I have [applied TCP pads / prepared the defibrillator / placed IV access].

9.7 RRT Documentation — Time-Stamped Record

The RRT documentation record serves three purposes: it provides a real-time record of interventions for the care team, it creates a handoff document for the receiving ICU team if the patient is transferred, and it provides the data source for hospital quality improvement and mortality review. The documentation should be completed in real time — not reconstructed from memory after the event.

REQUIRED RRT DOCUMENTATION ELEMENTS:

1. Time of RRT activation call: exact time the RRT was paged or called, and the name of the calling nurse.

2. Time of RRT arrival at bedside.

3. Initial assessment findings at time of arrival: HR, BP, SpO_2, RR, GCS or level of consciousness, rhythm and rate on the monitor, QRS width, any ST changes visible.

4. Rhythm strip at time of arrival: attach or reference the rhythm strip with the time printed. This is the baseline for comparison at each subsequent assessment.

5. Interventions: each medication (drug, dose, route, time, who administered), each electrical intervention (cardioversion/TCP: energy, SYNC status, result), each procedure (IV access, airway).

6. Physician notification: name, time, verbal response, orders received.

7. Patient response to each intervention: rhythm and hemodynamics at 2-minute intervals after each intervention.

8. Disposition: patient remains on unit with monitoring changes, transferred to ICU (time, receiving team), or Code Blue called (time, code team arrival).

BEDSIDE PEARL The most important RRT habit: call early, call for the rhythm. The RRT exists to prevent cardiac arrest — not to manage it once it has occurred. The bedside nurse who calls the RRT for a new Mobitz II in an asymptomatic patient is using the system exactly as intended. The nurse who waits until the patient's BP drops to 70/40 has allowed a preventable deterioration. When the telemetry shows a rhythm that requires immediate electrical intervention (TCP, cardioversion) or a rhythm that carries imminent VF risk (sustained VT, pre-excited AF, Mobitz II), the RRT call and the rhythm finding happen at the same moment — not after the next vital sign assessment or after the physician is reached.

KEY POINTS — CHAPTER 9

ECG-Triggered RRT Criteria

- Call the RRT for: new Mobitz II (even asymptomatic), new complete AV block with wide escape, sustained VT > 30 seconds, wide + irregular + > 200 bpm (pre-excited AF), electrical alternans + low voltage (tamponade), organized rhythm in unresponsive patient (possible PEA).
- Do not wait for symptoms or BP drop for Mobitz II or wide-escape complete AV block. The ECG finding alone is the activation criterion.

First 120 Seconds

- One voice, one leader. Arrive → Assess (look at patient, monitor, numbers) → Announce (state the finding) → Act (first intervention) → Delegate (assign tasks). Reassess every 2 minutes.

Bradycardia and Tachycardia Algorithms

- Bradycardia: narrow QRS = atropine first. Wide QRS = TCP immediately, no atropine. QRS width is the only decision point.
- Tachycardia: four branches from two binary decisions (QRS width + stability). Wide + unstable = synchronized cardioversion 100 J. Wide + polymorphic or pulseless = unsynchronized 200 J. Never verapamil/diltiazem for wide-complex tachycardia.

REMEMBER THIS

✓ The QRS width determines the first bradycardia intervention — always. Narrow QRS = atropine (AV-node-level, responds to vagolytic therapy). Wide QRS = TCP immediately (infranodal, no vagal innervation, atropine will not work). Giving atropine to a wide-escape bradycardia wastes the most critical minutes of the event while the patient continues at 28 bpm. Assess QRS width before reaching for atropine on every bradycardia RRT.

✓ Pre-excited AF is the tachycardia that does not fit the four-branch algorithm. Wide + irregular + > 200 bpm in a WPW patient is not 'wide-complex tachycardia' managed by the standard wide-QRS tachycardia branch. It requires procainamide (stable) or unsynchronized defibrillation (unstable), and it has an absolute contraindication list (adenosine, verapamil, diltiazem, digoxin, IV beta-blockers) that must be identified before any medication is given. Recognize the pattern before the medication cart is opened.

✓ Call the RRT before the patient deteriorates, not after. A new Mobitz II on the telemetry monitor at 2 AM in an asymptomatic patient with a BP of 118/74 is an RRT call. The patient who has Mobitz II progress to complete AV block with a wide ventricular escape at 28 bpm and a BP of 62/38 at 2:15 AM is a more difficult RRT call with a worse outcome. The 15 minutes between those two moments is the window that the RRT program exists to capture.

Special Populations — Pregnancy, Pediatrics & Elderly

When normal ranges are different and usual rules don't apply

ER NURSING · ICU NURSING · NCLEX

Three patient populations routinely produce ECG findings that do not match the standard adult reference ranges taught in Books 1 through 4 — and where applying standard adult management criteria without modification produces incorrect and potentially harmful decisions. The pregnant patient has a physiologically altered cardiovascular system that changes both the ECG baseline and the ACLS algorithm. The pediatric patient has age-specific normal ranges for every ECG parameter that differ dramatically from adult values. The elderly patient has a complex interaction of structural heart disease, polypharmacy, and autonomic changes that alters both the ECG presentation of arrhythmias and the safety profile of standard interventions.

Each section in this chapter first defines what is normal for the population, then identifies the most common errors that result from applying adult standard values to that population, and finally provides the modified management principles specific to each group.

10.1 Pregnancy — Normal ECG Changes

Pregnancy produces significant cardiovascular physiological changes that begin as early as the first trimester and peak in the third trimester. Many of these changes produce ECG findings that would be concerning in a non-pregnant patient but are entirely expected and benign in the pregnant patient. Recognizing these normal changes prevents unnecessary investigation and intervention.

ECG Finding in Pregnancy	Physiological Mechanism	Clinical Significance

Sinus tachycardia (HR 90-110 bpm)	Plasma volume expands by 40-50% in pregnancy, cardiac output increases 30-50%, and resting HR rises 10-20 bpm above the pre-pregnancy baseline.	Expected and normal throughout the second and third trimesters. Do not treat sinus tachycardia in pregnancy with rate-controlling agents unless the rate exceeds 150 bpm or there is a documented arrhythmia causing the tachycardia.
Left axis deviation (-15° to -30°)	The growing uterus displaces the diaphragm upward, which rotates the heart leftward and superiorly within the thoracic cavity.	Normal in pregnancy, particularly in the third trimester. Does not indicate pathological left axis deviation in this context. Compare to prior ECGs if available.
Q waves in III and aVF (small, < 0.04 s duration)	Same mechanism as the axis shift — cardiac rotation produces small Q waves in the inferior leads that were not present pre-pregnancy.	Normal in pregnancy. Must not be mistaken for pathological Q waves of prior inferior MI. Key distinguishing features: Q wave duration < 0.04 s, no associated ST or T wave changes, no ischemic symptoms.
Flattened or inverted T waves in leads III and V1-V3	Increased plasma volume and cardiac rotation alter repolarization vectors. T wave changes are common in leads that are perpendicular to the altered cardiac position.	Expected and non-specific in pregnancy. Do not diagnose ischemia based on T wave changes alone in a pregnant patient with no symptoms. Correlate with clinical presentation.

ST depression ≤ 1 mm (non-specific)	Volume-related changes in myocardial loading conditions alter repolarization. Mild non-specific ST depression can appear particularly in the third trimester.	Below 1 mm and without clinical correlation: normal. ST depression ≥ 1.5-2 mm or in a regional distribution requires the same evaluation as in any patient with possible ischemia.
Ectopic beats (PACs, PVCs)	Increased adrenergic tone and plasma volume expansion increase myocardial irritability in pregnancy.	Common, usually benign. Symptomatic palpitations are the most frequent cardiac complaint in pregnant patients and are usually from ectopy. Holter monitoring to document the arrhythmia is appropriate before any pharmacological intervention.

10.2 Cardiac Arrest in Pregnancy — Modified ACLS

Cardiac arrest in pregnancy is one of the most complex resuscitation scenarios in clinical practice. The gravid uterus compresses the inferior vena cava in the supine position, reducing venous return and cardiac output by up to 30% during CPR. Standard ACLS must be modified to address this compression, the fetal circulation, and the perimortem cesarean delivery decision.

CARDIAC ARREST IN PREGNANCY — MODIFIED ACLS SEQUENCE:

1. IMMEDIATE: Left uterine displacement (LUD) — manually push the uterus to the left with one or two hands, or tilt the patient 15-30° to the left using a wedge or folded blankets under the right hip. LUD must be maintained continuously throughout CPR. This single intervention can increase cardiac output during CPR by 20-30% by relieving IVC compression.

2. CPR: standard hand position (lower half of sternum) and depth (5-6 cm). The enlarged uterus raises the diaphragm and shifts abdominal contents, but the sternum position and compression mechanics remain the same. No modification to compression rate (100-120 per minute).

3. DEFIBRILLATION: same energy levels as standard ACLS (200 J biphasic for VF). Defibrillation is safe in pregnancy — do not delay or withhold defibrillation based on concern for fetal harm. The fetus receives a negligible current from standard defibrillation energy.

4. MEDICATIONS: same drugs, same doses as standard ACLS (epinephrine 1 mg IV/IO every 3-5 minutes, amiodarone 300 mg after 3rd shock). No medication modifications required for the arrest algorithm itself.

5. PERIMORTEM CESAREAN DELIVERY (PMCD): if ROSC is not achieved within 4 minutes of arrest, prepare for immediate PMCD. Delivery should be completed by 5 minutes from the time of arrest (the '4-minute rule'). PMCD improves both maternal and fetal outcomes: (a) removing the uterus eliminates IVC compression and dramatically improves maternal hemodynamics, and (b) the fetus can be resuscitated separately by the neonatal team. PMCD can be performed at the bedside without moving the patient.

6. POST-ROSC: if ROSC occurs, continue LUD. Targeted temperature management may be considered but should be planned with obstetrics consultation — maternal hypothermia affects fetal physiology. Emergent obstetric and maternal-fetal medicine consultation.

THE 4-MINUTE RULE: If ROSC has not been achieved within 4 minutes of cardiac arrest in a pregnancy ≥ 20 weeks gestation, prepare for perimortem cesarean delivery to be completed by 5 minutes. This guideline does not mean the mother is being given up on — PMCD often improves maternal hemodynamics enough to allow ROSC after delivery. The operation and the maternal resuscitation continue simultaneously.

10.3 Pediatric ECG — What Is Normal

The pediatric ECG cannot be read using adult reference ranges. Heart rate, QRS duration, PR interval, QTc, and axis all have age-specific normal values that differ substantially from adult norms, particularly in neonates and infants. Applying adult thresholds to a pediatric ECG will produce both false diagnoses (labeling normal as abnormal) and missed diagnoses (labeling abnormal as normal).

Parameter	Neonate (0-1 mo)	Infant (1-12 mo)	Child (1-8 yr)	Adult Reference
HR (bpm)	100-180	80-160	70-130	60-100
PR interval (s)	0.08-0.12	0.08-0.13	0.10-0.16	0.12-0.20
QRS duration (s)	0.04-0.08	0.04-0.08	0.06-0.09	0.06-0.10
QTc (s)	< 0.45	< 0.44	< 0.44	< 0.44 (M) < 0.45 (F)
QRS axis	+60° to +180°	+10° to +125°	+10° to +110°	-30° to +90°
R/S ratio in V1	R > S (normal)	R > S (normal)	R < S (normal)	R < S (normal)

Key Pediatric ECG Features That Differ from Adults

- R > S in V1 is NORMAL in neonates and infants: this pattern would suggest RVH in an adult but is the expected baseline in young children because the neonatal RV is proportionally larger than the LV at birth (both ventricles face the same pressure load in fetal circulation). The R/S ratio in V1 gradually reverses as the LV takes over pressure work after birth, reaching the adult pattern by age 3-5 years.
- Right axis deviation is NORMAL in neonates: an axis of +180° in a neonate is expected. The same axis in an adult indicates severe right heart disease. Use age-specific axis ranges.
- T waves: in the first week of life, T waves are upright in V1. After the first week and until puberty, T waves in V1 should be

negative. Upright T waves in V1 in a child between 1 week and puberty suggest RVH.

- HR: a heart rate of 140 bpm in a neonate is normal. The same rate in an adult requires evaluation for tachyarrhythmia. Pediatric SVT rates are often 220-300 bpm — significantly faster than adult SVT.
- QRS duration: pediatric QRS complexes are normally narrower than adult QRS complexes. A QRS of 0.10 s that is at the upper limit of normal for an adult is frankly wide for an infant.

10.4 Pediatric SVT — Recognition and Management

Supraventricular tachycardia is the most common sustained arrhythmia requiring treatment in children. It presents at rates that are dramatically faster than adult SVT (220-300 bpm in infants, compared to 140-220 bpm in adults) and produces hemodynamic instability more rapidly because of the infant's higher heart-rate dependence for maintaining cardiac output.

Feature	Pediatric SVT Details
Rate	220-300 bpm in infants. 180-240 bpm in older children. The very fast rate distinguishes SVT from sinus tachycardia (which is usually ≤ 220 bpm even in a very sick infant). An abrupt onset and offset (not gradual) also distinguishes SVT from sinus tachycardia.
ECG appearance	Regular narrow-complex tachycardia at the above rates. P waves may not be visible or may appear as a retrograde P wave after the QRS. The absence of visible P waves at very fast rates is expected.
Vagal maneuvers (first-line, all ages)	Infant: ice bag applied to the face for 10-15 seconds (dive reflex — extremely effective in infants). Older child: Valsalva maneuver, carotid sinus massage (avoid in children with known cervical pathology). Modified Valsalva (supine, blow into syringe, then leg raise) is effective in children as in adults.

Adenosine (second-line if vagal fails)	Dose: 0.1 mg/kg rapid IV push (maximum first dose 6 mg). Second dose if needed: 0.2 mg/kg (maximum 12 mg). Same rapid-push + saline flush technique as adults. The proximal IV site requirement is the same — distal hand or foot IV leads to adenosine degradation before reaching the AV node.
Synchronized cardioversion (unstable)	Energy: 0.5-1 J/kg biphasic synchronized first attempt. If unsuccessful: 2 J/kg. Pediatric defibrillation pads (smaller size) should be used for children < 10 kg — do not use adult pads on infants.

PEDIATRIC DOSE ERRORS: Adenosine and defibrillation energy in children are weight-based. Never administer adult doses to a child. Use the Broselow tape (length-based weight estimation) to estimate weight if it is not known. If Broselow is unavailable: ask the parent or caregiver for the child's most recent weight in kg. Document the estimated weight used for dose calculation in the chart. Overdose of adenosine in a child produces prolonged AV block and can cause several seconds of asystole that is frightening but usually self-terminating.

10.5 Elderly-Specific Arrhythmia Patterns

The elderly cardiac patient differs from the standard adult ECG population in three important ways: structural changes (fibrosis, amyloid deposition, valve disease, and coronary disease alter the myocardium in ways that change normal ECG parameters), autonomic changes (reduced baroreceptor sensitivity, reduced sympathetic responsiveness, and blunted vagal responses alter the arrhythmia presentation), and polypharmacy (the drug burden of managing multiple chronic conditions creates a high baseline QTc-prolonging and AV-conduction-slowing medication load).

Elderly-Specific Pattern	Clinical Significance and Modified Management

Sick sinus syndrome (SSS) with tachy-brady pattern	The most common indication for permanent pacemaker in the elderly. ECG: alternating periods of sinus bradycardia or pauses and bursts of atrial tachyarrhythmia (AF, flutter, or atrial tachycardia). The bradycardia is intrinsic SA node dysfunction; the tachycardia is the reflex atrial response. Management: permanent pacemaker (usually dual-chamber, DDD) to manage the bradycardia, then safe rate-controlling or antiarrhythmic agents can be used for the tachycardia component without risk of worsening the bradycardia.
Chronic atrial fibrillation with variable ventricular rate	Most elderly patients with AF have been in the rhythm for months to years. The management goal is rate control (not rhythm control in most), anticoagulation per CHA_2DS_2-VASc scoring, and symptom management. Cardioversion in chronic AF without anticoagulation coverage or TEE to exclude LAA thrombus carries a high stroke risk.
Left bundle branch block (often chronic)	New LBBB in an elderly patient with chest pain requires Sgarbossa criteria (Book 3, Chapter 6). Chronic LBBB that has been present on multiple prior ECGs is a baseline finding, not an emergency in isolation. Always obtain prior ECGs before labeling LBBB as 'new.'
PR prolongation and AV block	Age-related fibrosis of the conduction system produces progressive AV block at a rate of approximately 1% per decade after age 60. First-degree AV block is common and benign. Wenckebach may represent age-related fibrosis rather than acute ischemia. Complete AV block from fibrosis (Lenegre disease) requires permanent pacemaker.
QT prolongation from polypharmacy	The elderly patient's medication list commonly includes two to four QTc-prolonging agents simultaneously. Age-related renal and hepatic clearance reduction amplifies the QTc effect of each drug. QTc monitoring every 24-48 hours is appropriate for any elderly ICU patient on QTc-prolonging medications.

10.6 Drug Dosing and QT in the Elderly

The QTc risk in elderly patients is amplified by multiple concurrent factors that are each independently dangerous but together produce a substantially higher torsades risk than any single factor would predict. Managing this risk requires a systematic medication review at every care transition: admission, transfer, and discharge.

- Renal clearance decline: creatinine clearance decreases progressively with age even when the serum creatinine appears normal (because muscle mass also declines with age, producing a falsely reassuring creatinine). Renally cleared drugs — including sotalol, digoxin, and many antibiotics — accumulate to higher plasma levels in the elderly at standard doses. Always calculate eGFR using a validated formula (CKD-EPI or Cockcroft-Gault) rather than using the serum creatinine alone.
- Hepatic clearance decline: hepatic first-pass metabolism and cytochrome P450 activity decline with age. Hepatically cleared QTc-prolonging drugs (amiodarone, some antifungals, diltiazem) have prolonged half-lives in the elderly. QTc prolongation from amiodarone is amplified in elderly patients, particularly those with low body weight.
- Drug interactions: polypharmacy increases the probability of CYP450-mediated drug interactions that raise plasma levels of QTc-prolonging drugs to toxic ranges. Common interactions: azole antifungals (fluconazole, voriconazole) inhibit CYP3A4, raising plasma levels of many drugs including methadone and some antipsychotics.
- Electrolyte vulnerability: elderly patients are more prone to both hypokalemia (diuretic therapy is more common) and hypomagnesemia (loop diuretics, poor dietary intake). The combination of polypharmacy QTc risk and electrolyte instability creates a high-risk substrate.
- Practical threshold: in the elderly ICU patient, target K^+ ≥4.5 mEq/L (slightly higher than the standard 4.0 target) and Mg^{2+} ≥2.0 mEq/L when any QTc-prolonging medication is on the medication list. Review and reduce the QTc medication burden at every care transition.

10.7 End-of-Life ECG Patterns

The care of patients at the end of life includes managing cardiac monitoring in a way that is consistent with the patient's goals of care. In patients who have elected comfort-focused care or have a do-not-resuscitate (DNR) order, certain ECG findings have a different clinical significance than they would in a patient for whom full resuscitation is the plan. This section addresses the specific ECG patterns that are most commonly encountered in the end-of-life setting.

ECG Pattern	End-of-Life Context and Nursing Role
Agonal rhythm (wide, slow, irregular QRS complexes at < 20 bpm)	Agonal rhythms represent the final electrical activity of a dying heart. They are not a rhythm that can be treated effectively — defibrillation and cardiac medications do not restore meaningful cardiac function from an agonal rhythm in a patient whose underlying disease process has produced irreversible multi-organ failure. Document the rhythm, document the time of onset, and notify the physician. If DNR: no resuscitation interventions. Comfort measures (positioning, oral care, pain and symptom management) are the clinical priority.
Sinus bradycardia with progressive PR lengthening	A common terminal rhythm pattern: the sinus rate slows progressively, the PR interval lengthens, and eventually AV block and then asystole follow. In a comfort-focused patient, this progression is expected and does not require intervention. Maintain the patient's comfort and notify the family that the rhythm changes indicate the patient is approaching death.
Asystole (flat line)	Confirmed absence of cardiac electrical activity in a patient with an active DNR order requires: (1) confirmation of asystole in at least two leads, (2) notation of the time, (3) physician notification, (4) no CPR or resuscitation measures. Document the time and lead confirmation in the chart.

Persistent monitoring in DNR patients	The question of whether to continue cardiac monitoring in a comfort-focused patient should be addressed at care planning. Continuous monitoring of a DNR patient who is actively dying can create distress for the family if every alarm is audible. Consider whether discontinuing monitoring is consistent with the patient's goals of care and discuss with the family and team.

DNR AND MONITORING: A DNR order does not mean 'do not monitor' and does not mean 'do not treat.' DNR means do not perform cardiopulmonary resuscitation (chest compressions, defibrillation, and advanced airway management) in the event of cardiac arrest. All other nursing care, monitoring, and medical interventions remain appropriate unless additional restrictions (DNI, DNH, comfort-measures-only) have been specified in the patient's advance directive or orders. Clarify the scope of the DNR with the physician and document the discussion.

BEDSIDE PEARL The three populations in this chapter share one clinical principle: normal is not universal. A sinus rate of 140 bpm means something fundamentally different in a neonate (normal), a pregnant woman in the third trimester (mildly elevated but possibly normal), and an elderly patient with no prior cardiac history (requires evaluation). The ECG interpretation skill that transfers across all three populations is the same: compare to the appropriate reference range for the specific patient in front of you, not the adult normal table on the wall.

KEY POINTS — CHAPTER 10

Pregnancy

- Normal pregnancy ECG changes: sinus tachycardia (90-110 bpm), left axis deviation, small Q waves in III/aVF, non-specific ST-T changes, PACs/PVCs. None require treatment in isolation in an asymptomatic patient.
- Cardiac arrest in pregnancy: LUD immediately and continuously, PMCD by 5 minutes if no ROSC, same

defibrillation energy, same medications. Defibrillation is safe for the fetus.

Pediatrics

- Age-specific normal ranges: neonate HR 100-180, R > S in V1 is normal until age 3-5, right axis is normal in neonates. Apply age-specific tables, not adult values.
- Pediatric SVT: 220-300 bpm in infants. Vagal first (ice to face in infants), then adenosine 0.1 mg/kg (max 6 mg first dose). Cardioversion 0.5-1 J/kg. All doses weight-based — use Broselow tape.

Elderly

- SSS tachy-brady pattern: permanent pacemaker first, then safe antiarrhythmics for tachycardia. Chronic AF: rate control + anticoagulation (CHA_2DS_2-VASc). Chronic LBBB: always compare to prior ECG before calling it new.
- QTc risk: renal and hepatic clearance decline amplifies drug QTc effects. Target K^+ ≥4.5 and Mg^{2+} ≥2.0 in elderly patients on QTc-prolonging medications. Calculate eGFR, not just serum creatinine.

REMEMBER THIS

✓ Pregnancy ACLS: left uterine displacement from the first second of CPR, maintained continuously. This single intervention restores 20-30% of the cardiac output lost from IVC compression by the gravid uterus. LUD must be maintained by a dedicated team member throughout the resuscitation. Perimortem cesarean delivery at 4 minutes if no ROSC — this is not abandoning the mother. It is the intervention most likely to allow ROSC.

✓ Pediatric ECG values are not adult ECG values with smaller numbers. R > S in V1 is normal in a neonate and abnormal in an adult. A heart rate of 160 bpm is normal in a neonate and requires evaluation in an adult. An axis of +150° is normal in a neonate and indicates severe right heart disease in an adult. Use the age-specific table for every pediatric ECG parameter. The adult reference table does not apply.

✓ The elderly patient's QTc risk is not just about the current medication list — it is about the cumulative effect of impaired renal and hepatic clearance on every drug the patient has been taking for years. The drug that is at a safe dose in a 40-year-old with normal renal function may be at a toxic level in an 80-year-old with eGFR 32. Calculate the eGFR, review every QTc-prolonging drug, and set the electrolyte targets slightly higher (K^+ ≥4.5, not just 4.0) in the elderly ICU patient.

Telemetry Communication & Escalation

What to say, when to say it, and how to document it

ER NURSING · ICU NURSING · RAPID RESPONSE

Every skill in this book ends the same way: a communication. The ECG finding matters only if the right person receives the right information at the right time and takes the right action. A nurse who recognizes a Wellens pattern, a new Mobitz II, or a pre-excited AF but cannot communicate that finding clearly — or whose communication is not documented — has completed only half of the clinical task.

This chapter provides the specific communication frameworks, escalation pathways, and documentation standards that transform ECG recognition skills into patient outcomes. The SBAR templates, read-back protocols, chain-of-escalation decision tree, and handoff communication guide are all designed to be used directly at the bedside, not as theoretical frameworks.

11.1 SBAR for Arrhythmia Calls — Six Scenario Templates

The SBAR format (Situation, Background, Assessment, Recommendation) is the standard communication structure for clinical handoffs and urgent notifications in healthcare. The following six templates cover the most common arrhythmia communication scenarios. Each is designed to be delivered in under 60 seconds, providing the receiving provider with every critical fact needed to make a management decision.

SCENARIO 1: NEW VT ON TELEMETRY (STABLE PATIENT)

S — Situation: This is [Name], RN on [Unit], calling about [Patient Name] in Room [X]. The patient has a new wide-complex regular tachycardia on the monitor at [rate] bpm.

B — Background: The patient is [age, sex, primary diagnosis]. Current vitals: HR [X], BP [X], SpO_2 [X]%. The patient is [alert and responding / mentating normally]. The wide-complex tachycardia started at [time] and has been present for [X] minutes. Prior rhythm was [sinus / AF / other]. IV access is established.

A — Assessment: I am concerned this is ventricular tachycardia. The patient is currently hemodynamically stable but the rhythm is wide, regular, and faster than [prior rate]. Brugada criteria [have been applied / are pending physician review].

R — Recommendation: I need a physician at the bedside immediately. I am preparing IV amiodarone 150 mg per the stable VT protocol and have placed defibrillation pads on the patient. Please advise on medication initiation.

SCENARIO 2: INFERIOR STEMI WITH V4R POSITIVE

S — Situation: This is [Name], RN, calling about [Patient Name] in Room [X]. The patient has a 12-lead ECG showing inferior STEMI and a positive V4R. I am requesting STEMI protocol activation.

B — Background: The patient is [age, sex] presenting with crushing chest pain for [X] minutes. Vitals: HR [X], BP [X], SpO_2 [X]%. The 12-lead shows ST elevation in II, III, aVF ([X] mm each) with reciprocal depression in I and aVL. V4R was obtained at [time] and shows [X] mm ST elevation confirming RV infarction.

A — Assessment: This is an inferior STEMI with RV infarction. Nitroglycerin and morphine are being held. The patient is [hemodynamically stable / hypotensive — IV fluid bolus initiated].

R — Recommendation: I am requesting immediate STEMI protocol activation and physician assessment at the bedside. I have [aspirin given / IV access in place / patient NPO]. Please confirm cath lab activation.

SCENARIO 3: HIGH-RISK PATTERN — WELLENS / DE WINTER / LEFT MAIN

S — Situation: This is [Name], RN, calling about [Patient Name] in Room [X]. I have identified a high-risk ECG pattern that requires urgent physician review.

B — Background: The patient is [age, sex, diagnosis]. The ECG obtained at [time] shows [deep symmetric T wave inversions V2-V3 consistent with Wellens syndrome / upsloping ST depression with tall peaked T waves V1-V4 consistent with de Winter pattern / diffuse ST depression in [X] leads with ST elevation in aVR consistent with left main disease]. The patient [is pain-free and appears comfortable / has ongoing chest pain].

A — Assessment: I am concerned this pattern indicates [critical proximal LAD stenosis that requires urgent angiography / acute LAD occlusion requiring STEMI-equivalent activation / left main disease requiring urgent angiography]. [If Wellens: I am not proceeding with the ordered stress test until this is reviewed.]

R — Recommendation: I need a physician to review this ECG at the bedside immediately. [If Wellens: I am placing the patient NPO and cancelling the stress test order pending your review.] Please advise on disposition and whether cardiology consultation is required now.

SCENARIO 4: COMPLETE AV BLOCK WITH WIDE ESCAPE

S — Situation: This is [Name], RN on [Unit], calling about [Patient Name] in Room [X]. The patient has developed complete AV block with a slow wide ventricular escape rhythm.

B — Background: The patient is [age, sex, diagnosis]. Current vitals: HR [X] (ventricular escape rate), BP [X], SpO_2 [X]%. The monitor shows P waves at [X] bpm with no relationship to QRS complexes, and a wide QRS escape rhythm at [X] bpm. IV access is established. The patient is [conscious / altered].

A — Assessment: This is complete AV block with wide ventricular escape at [X] bpm. The wide QRS indicates infranodal block. Atropine will not be effective. I am concerned about hemodynamic instability.

R — Recommendation: I am applying transcutaneous pacing pads now and requesting physician assessment at the bedside immediately. Please provide orders for TCP initiation parameters and analgesia. I am also notifying the charge nurse.

SCENARIO 5: PRE-EXCITED AF — HOLDING ORDERED MEDICATION

S — Situation: This is [Name], RN, calling to report a medication safety concern for [Patient Name] in Room [X]. I am holding the ordered [diltiazem / verapamil / adenosine] and requesting an urgent physician review.

B — Background: The patient has a known WPW history [or: has a baseline ECG showing short PR and delta waves]. The current rhythm is a wide, irregular tachycardia at [X] bpm. This pattern is consistent with pre-excited AF. The ordered [diltiazem / adenosine] is an AV-nodal blocking agent.

A — Assessment: Administering [diltiazem / adenosine] to a patient with pre-excited AF can produce ventricular rates exceeding 300 bpm and trigger ventricular fibrillation. This is an absolute contraindication in this rhythm.

R — Recommendation: I am holding the [medication] order and requesting physician assessment at the bedside immediately. The correct management for stable pre-excited AF is IV procainamide. For unstable: immediate unsynchronized defibrillation. Please advise and revise the orders.

SCENARIO 6: QTc > 0.50 s IN AN ICU PATIENT

S — Situation: This is [Name], RN in the ICU, calling about [Patient Name]. The patient's QTc has increased to [X] s on the most recent 12-lead ECG.

B — Background: The patient is on [list QTc-prolonging medications]. Current electrolytes: K^+ [X] mEq/L, Mg^{2+} [X] mEq/L. The baseline QTc on admission was [X] s. Today's QTc is [X] s — a change of [X] s from baseline. The [medication] was started [X] days ago.

A — Assessment: The QTc is now above the 0.50 s threshold for high torsades risk. With the current electrolytes and medication burden, I am concerned about the risk of torsades de pointes.

R — Recommendation: I am requesting a physician review of the current medication list and electrolyte targets. I have [already begun K^+ and Mg^{2+} repletion / am requesting orders for electrolyte repletion]. The defibrillator is at the bedside. Please advise on whether any QTc-prolonging medications should be held or substituted.

11.2 Read-Back and Closed-Loop Communication

Closed-loop communication is the process by which a receiver confirms receipt and understanding of a message by repeating it back to the sender. In arrhythmia management, closed-loop communication is particularly important because the consequences of a misheard order or a miscommunicated finding can be immediately life-threatening.

Situation	Closed-Loop Communication Standard
Receiving a verbal medication order during a cardiac event	Read back the order immediately: 'I am reading back: amiodarone 150 mg IV over 10 minutes — is that correct?' Wait for explicit confirmation from the ordering provider before administering. Do not proceed on a verbal order that has not been confirmed.
Receiving a STEMI protocol activation confirmation	'Confirming: you are activating the STEMI protocol for [patient name], Room [X], and the cath lab is being notified now — is that correct?' Document the confirmation and the time in the chart.
Communicating a medication hold	After holding a medication and notifying the physician: 'Confirming you are aware I am holding the [medication] for [patient name] due to [reason], and you will provide an alternative order — is that correct?' Do not consider the communication complete until the physician has verbally confirmed awareness.
Handoff of a patient with an ongoing rhythm issue	'I am transferring care of [patient] to [name]. The current rhythm is [X], the last event was at [time], the current orders are [X], and the next reassessment is due at [time]. Do you have any questions or concerns?' Wait for confirmation that the receiving nurse has understood all critical elements.

DOCUMENTATION OF VERBAL ORDERS: All verbal orders received during a cardiac emergency must be documented with: (1) the exact order as received, (2) the name of the ordering provider, (3) the time the order was received, and (4) the read-back confirmation. Verbal orders must be co-signed by the ordering provider within the institutional timeframe (typically 24 hours). During a code or RRT event, a designated documenter should be assigned specifically to record verbal orders in real time.

11.3 Chain of Escalation — When to Move to the Next Level

The chain of escalation defines who to call, in what order, and under what circumstances when a clinical situation is not being adequately addressed through the standard communication pathway. In the cardiac monitoring context, escalation is required when: the patient's condition is deteriorating and the current response is insufficient, a provider has not responded to a notification within an appropriate timeframe, or a medication order has been given that the nurse believes is contraindicated.

Level	Contact	When to Escalate to This Level
1	**Bedside physician or hospitalist covering the unit**	First call for any new significant finding: new arrhythmia, STEMI pattern, high-risk ECG pattern, QTc > 0.50 s, medication safety concern. Expected response: physician at the bedside or phone orders within 10-15 minutes for urgent findings, 30 minutes for non-urgent findings.
2	**Charge nurse or senior nurse supervisor**	If the covering physician has not responded within the expected timeframe, or if the nurse's clinical concern is not being adequately addressed by the initial provider response. The charge nurse can facilitate communication and escalation and can involve the house supervisor if needed.
3	**Cardiology consult (attending or fellow on call)**	For rhythm-specific expertise: new sustained VT not responding to amiodarone, new complete AV block requiring pacemaker evaluation, Wellens or de Winter pattern not being acted on as a STEMI-equivalent, pre-excited AF where the covering physician is uncertain of management.

4	**Rapid Response Team (RRT)**	If the patient is deteriorating and the current management is insufficient, or if the nurse cannot reach the responsible physician within an urgent timeframe and the patient's condition requires immediate intervention. The RRT call bypasses the normal chain and brings a multidisciplinary team to the bedside immediately.
5	**Code Blue**	Cardiac arrest (pulseless, unresponsive, or confirmed VF/pulseless VT). Activates the full resuscitation team. Does not require prior RRT activation or physician notification.

ESCALATION IS NOT INSUBORDINATION: A nurse who escalates a clinical concern through the chain of command when an initial provider response is inadequate is fulfilling a professional and ethical obligation, not challenging authority. The Joint Commission and the ANA Nursing Standards both explicitly require nurses to escalate when they believe patient safety is at risk and initial communication has not produced an adequate response. Document every escalation attempt: who was contacted, at what time, what was communicated, and what response was received.

11.4 Documentation Sequence — What the Chart Must Show

The documentation sequence for a significant arrhythmia event must be completed in real time, not reconstructed from memory after the event. Retrospective documentation is less reliable, is flagged as such by chart audit systems, and provides less legal protection than contemporaneous entries. The following sequence covers the minimum documentation standard for any significant cardiac monitoring finding.

ARRHYTHMIA EVENT DOCUMENTATION SEQUENCE:

1. Time of finding identification: the exact clock time the rhythm change or alarm was first noted. This is the starting point of the documentation record.

2. ECG or rhythm finding description: rate, rhythm name or description, QRS width (narrow or wide), regularity (regular or irregular), any ST changes (lead, mm, direction). E.g., 'At 02:14, monitor shows regular wide-complex tachycardia at 162 bpm, QRS 0.16 s.'

3. Clinical assessment at the time of finding: patient's level of consciousness, response to voice, vital signs (HR, BP, SpO_2, RR), presence or absence of symptoms (chest pain, dyspnea, palpitations). E.g., 'Patient alert and diaphoretic, BP 88/50, SpO_2 96% on room air, reporting palpitations and mild dyspnea.'

4. Action taken: specific intervention initiated at the bedside before provider contact. E.g., 'Defibrillation pads applied. IV access confirmed patent. 12-lead ECG obtained at 02:16.'

5. Provider notification: provider name, title, method of contact (phone/bedside), exact time of notification, and the key information communicated. E.g., 'Dr. [Name] notified by phone at 02:17. SBAR communicated: new wide-complex tachycardia at 162 bpm, BP 88/50, hemodynamically compromised, request for bedside assessment.'

6. Orders received: each order with drug name, dose, route, and time received. E.g., 'Order received at 02:18: amiodarone 150 mg IV over 10 minutes. Verbal order read back and confirmed by Dr. [Name].'

7. Interventions administered: drug, dose, route, time administered, and who administered. E.g., 'Amiodarone 150 mg IV push over 10 minutes initiated at 02:19 by RN [Name].'

8. Patient response: vital signs and rhythm status at 5-10 minute intervals after intervention. E.g., 'At 02:30: rhythm converted to sinus rhythm at 88 bpm. BP improved to 108/70. Patient reports palpitations resolved. 12-lead ECG obtained.'

11.5 Handoff Communication — Nothing Gets Lost Between Shifts

Shift handoff is the highest-risk communication event in inpatient cardiac monitoring. Studies of adverse cardiac events consistently show that a disproportionate number occur in the hour immediately after a shift change, and that inadequate handoff communication is a contributing factor. The following handoff standard for cardiac monitoring patients addresses the specific ECG-related information that must be explicitly communicated — not assumed to be findable in the chart.

Handoff Element	Specific Content Required
Current rhythm and baseline	State the current rhythm by name (not just 'the heart rate is fine'). E.g., 'Patient is in sinus rhythm at 72 bpm, known LBBB, QRS 0.14 s — this is the patient's chronic baseline. Sgarbossa criteria would apply if chest pain recurs.' This ensures the receiving nurse knows what to compare to if the rhythm changes.
Any rhythm events during the shift	Every significant rhythm event from the outgoing shift: what happened, what time, what was done, and what the outcome was. E.g., 'At 02:14, new VT at 162 bpm. Amiodarone 150 mg given. Converted at 02:30. Now in sinus. Cardiology notified, amiodarone infusion running at 1 mg/min — check the bag volume.'
Active monitoring parameters	CSTM lead selection and current baseline values. QTc — the most recent value and the trend. Alarm thresholds — whether any have been customized from default and why. E.g., 'CSTM baseline in V5 is -0.2 mm. Notify me if it changes ±1 mm. QTc today was 0.49 s, up from 0.44 s admission. The QTc alarm is set at 0.50 s.'
Medications of cardiac concern	Any cardiac medications that were started, changed, or held during the shift. Specifically: QTc-prolonging agents added or dose-changed, antiarrhythmics started or infusing, medications held due to contraindication. E.g., 'Haloperidol was added at 22:00 for delirium. QTc should be rechecked at 06:00 — it's in the MAR as a nursing order.'
Outstanding provider notifications or pending orders	Any communication that occurred during the outgoing shift that the receiving nurse needs to follow up on. E.g., 'Cardiology was notified about the VT at 02:30. They plan to call back between 07:00-08:00 for a disposition decision. Chart note expected.'

Equipment and device status	Pacemaker-dependent patients: wire connections, current pacing settings, threshold last checked. Patients with temporary devices: TCP pads still in place from an earlier event (vs removed), defibrillator at bedside vs returned to hallway, epicardial wire status.

END-OF-SHIFT CARDIAC MONITORING CHECKLIST — COMPLETE BEFORE HANDING OFF:

1. Confirm current rhythm name and document it in the handoff note. Do not say 'looks normal' — name the rhythm.

2. Review the CSTM trend for the entire shift. Is there any unaddressed ST change from baseline? If yes, ensure it is documented and the receiving nurse is explicitly informed.

3. Check the current QTc. Is it above 0.44 s (women) or 0.43 s (men)? Above 0.50 s? Communicate the value and the trend to the receiving nurse.

4. Review the medication administration record: any QTc-prolonging drugs added this shift? Any cardiac drugs held with a pending clarification? Communicate specifically.

5. Confirm all provider notifications from the shift are documented with time, provider name, and response. Identify any outstanding follow-up expected in the next shift.

6. Confirm alarm thresholds are set appropriately for this patient's known baseline and that the receiving nurse understands why any non-default thresholds are in place.

7. For pacemaker patients: confirm pacing settings, check wire connections, verify capture on the last rhythm strip. Document the current pacing status in the handoff.

BEDSIDE PEARL The SBAR communication skill that separates effective from ineffective nursing practice in arrhythmia management is not the format — it is the specificity. A provider who receives the call 'the patient's heart rate is fast and I'm not sure what it is' cannot make a management decision from the other end of the phone. A provider who receives 'wide-complex regular tachycardia at 162 bpm, QRS 0.16 s, BP 88/50, patient diaphoretic, pads applied, requesting amiodarone order' has everything needed to make a decision in under 15 seconds. Practice stating the rhythm by its full name, the rate, the QRS width, the BP, and the stability assessment in one sentence. That sentence is the core of every arrhythmia SBAR, and it takes less than 10 seconds to deliver.

SBAR Communication

- Name the rhythm specifically — never 'the heart rate is off' or 'the rhythm looks funny.' State: rhythm name, rate, QRS width, BP, and stability in the first sentence of every arrhythmia SBAR call.
- Six templates cover the most common scenarios: stable VT, inferior STEMI + positive V4R, high-risk pattern (Wellens/de Winter/left main), complete AV block, pre-excited AF medication hold, and QTc > 0.50 s. Know the template for each before you need it.

Closed-Loop and Escalation

- Read back every verbal order before administering: state the drug, dose, and route and wait for explicit confirmation. Document the read-back in the chart.
- Escalation is a professional obligation, not insubordination. Document every escalation attempt with the provider name, time, communication content, and response. If the response is inadequate and the patient is deteriorating: activate the RRT without waiting for the next level to respond.

Documentation and Handoff

- Document in real time: time of finding, ECG description, clinical assessment, action, provider notification, orders, interventions, patient response. Never reconstruct from memory.
- Handoff must include: current rhythm by name, every rhythm event during the shift, CSTM baseline and QTc, cardiac medications changed or held, outstanding notifications, and pacemaker/device status. 'Looks normal' is not a handoff.

REMEMBER THIS

✓ The SBAR call works only if the Assessment component is specific. For arrhythmia calls: the assessment sentence should state your conclusion about the rhythm and the risk it poses. 'I believe this is ventricular tachycardia and the patient is hemodynamically compromised' gives the provider a specific clinical conclusion to agree or disagree with. 'I'm not sure what the rhythm is' requires the provider to make the assessment from a description alone without seeing the patient. Commit to the assessment, communicate it clearly, and document it.

✓ Closed-loop communication is not optional in high-stakes cardiac events. A verbal order that is not read back is an order that can be misheard, misremembered, or disputed. The read-back takes 5 seconds. The consequences of a missed or incorrect dose of amiodarone, adenosine, or procainamide in a cardiac emergency can be irreversible. Read every verbal order back, wait for confirmation, and document the confirmation.

✓ The highest-risk time window for a monitored cardiac patient is the 60 minutes after shift change. The handoff that names the rhythm, describes the shift's events, states the QTc value and trend, identifies all cardiac medication changes, and confirms alarm thresholds — that handoff creates a receiving nurse who is fully informed from the first minute of the shift. The handoff that ends with 'everything's fine' creates a receiving nurse who must rediscover the patient's cardiac situation from scratch.

Full Integration — The Bedside Read from Monitor to Action

Everything in Book 5 in one repeatable real-time method

ER NURSING · ICU NURSING · RAPID RESPONSE · ACLS

This is the chapter where everything in Book 5 becomes one repeatable sequence. Chapters 1 through 11 built the individual skills: the Big 5 triage scan, the Brugada algorithm, the V4R nitrate pause, the high-risk patterns, the tiered ICU alarm response, the cardiac surgery ECG framework, the metabolic drug management protocol, the hemodynamic-ECG integration, the RRT algorithms, the special population modifications, and the SBAR communication templates. This chapter integrates all of them into a single bedside method that can be run on any ECG, in any clinical setting, at any time.

The method has six phases. Each phase takes a defined amount of time and produces a specific output. The sequence does not vary based on the clinical setting, the patient population, or the apparent urgency of the presentation. The sequence that runs automatically in the most routine situation is the same sequence that runs in the most time-critical one.

12.1 The 10-Second Triage — Rate, Rhythm, ST

Before any systematic read begins, the first 10 seconds identify whether the patient requires an immediate intervention before the full method can be completed. This is the safety net that prevents the systematic read from delaying treatment in a cardiac arrest, a pulseless rhythm, or an immediately life-threatening arrhythmia.

10-SECOND TRIAGE — THREE QUESTIONS, ANSWER IN ORDER:

1. Is the patient PULSELESS? If the monitor shows any rhythm and the patient is unresponsive: confirm no pulse immediately. If pulseless: CPR and ACLS protocol. Do not proceed to Step 2.

2. Is there a LIFE-THREATENING RHYTHM on the monitor right now? VF (chaotic, no QRS), pulseless VT (wide regular, no pulse), or complete asystole (flat line confirmed in multiple leads): act on the rhythm immediately. Do not proceed to Step 3.
3. Is there any finding that requires action BEFORE the full systematic read? Wide-complex tachycardia with hemodynamic instability (synchronized cardioversion), bradycardia with hemodynamic instability (TCP if wide QRS, atropine if narrow QRS), or a recognizable high-risk pattern (Wellens, de Winter, pre-excited AF, electrical alternans): identify and communicate before completing the full read.

WHAT THE 10-SECOND TRIAGE IS NOT: It is not a replacement for the full 8-step method. Every patient who passes through the 10-second triage without triggering an immediate action still receives the full systematic read. The triage asks only one question: does something need to happen RIGHT NOW before the full read is complete? If the answer is no, the full method proceeds immediately.

12.2 The Full 8-Step Method Under Bedside Time Pressure

The 8-step reading method from Book 3 Chapter 12 is applied here with the bedside time constraints of an emergency department, ICU, or ward setting. The sequence is identical to the academic version, but the pace is compressed and each step is paired with the specific decision it triggers in real time.

Step	Assess	If Abnormal — Bedside Decision	Time Budget
1	**Rate and rhythm**	VF/pulseless VT → ACLS. Wide-complex tachycardia → stability assessment (Chapter 2). Bradycardia with compromise → QRS width decision (Chapter 9).	< 5 s

2	**Axis**	Unexpected new left axis → consider LAFB, prior inferior MI. Extreme right axis → acute RV strain, exclude PE.	5 s
3	**Intervals**	QRS > 0.12 s → STOP, go to Step 5 before reading ST. QTc > 0.50 s → notify provider, review medications, electrolytes.	10 s
4	**Chamber enlargement**	LVH criteria met → ST-T changes in Steps 6-7 may be strain (not ischemia). Flag before reading ST.	5 s
5	**QRS morphology / BBB**	LBBB or paced rhythm → SWITCH to Sgarbossa criteria for Steps 6-7. Do not apply standard STEMI thresholds.	10 s
6	**ST segment**	Standard criteria (no BBB): elevation with reciprocal → STEMI. Inferior elevation → V4R before nitrates. Diffuse depression + aVR elevation → left main urgency. Sgarbossa (BBB/paced): concordant elevation → STEMI-equivalent.	20 s

7	**T waves**	Deep symmetric V2-V3 inversions (pain-free) → Wellens. Upsloping ST depression + peaked T in V1-V4 → de Winter. Peaked tent-shaped T → hyperkalemia. QTU prolongation + flat T → hypokalemia.	15 s
8	**Clinical correlation**	Normal ECG + compelling story → serial ECGs + troponins, never discharge. ECG matches the story → act on the diagnosis. ECG does not match → consider lead reversal, artifact, mimic.	10 s

TOTAL SYSTEMATIC READ TIME: Steps 1-8 together take approximately 80 seconds on a straightforward ECG. A complex ECG with multiple findings may take 3-4 minutes. The time budget column above is a guide, not a rigid rule. The two steps that must never be skipped regardless of time pressure: Step 5 (BBB check before ST reading) and Step 8 (clinical correlation). These are the two steps where the most clinically dangerous errors occur.

12.3 The Five Branch Points

After the 8-step method, five diagnostic branch points must each be assessed before the ECG read is considered complete. Missing any one of them produces a gap in the interpretation that the next clinician to see the patient will have to fill — and may not fill correctly.

Branch Point	Question	If Yes — Action

Standard STEMI criteria	Is there regional ST elevation (≥1 mm limb, ≥2 mm precordial) in ≥2 contiguous leads, with a normal QRS?	STEMI protocol activation. V4R if inferior territory. Notify cath lab. Do not apply standard criteria if QRS is wide — go to Branch 2.
Sgarbossa / modified Sgarbossa	Is the QRS wide (≥0.12 s) from LBBB or paced rhythm?	Apply Sgarbossa criteria. Rule 1 (concordant ST elevation ≥1 mm in any lead) or Rule 2 (concordant ST depression ≥1 mm in V1-V3) = STEMI-equivalent. Rule 3: calculate ST elevation ÷ S-wave depth ≤ -0.25 in the most discordant lead.
Pericarditis differential	Is the ST elevation diffuse (most or all leads), concave, with PR depression and NO reciprocal depression?	Pericarditis — NSAIDs + colchicine, not cath lab. Serial ECGs for 4-stage evolution tracking. Do NOT activate STEMI protocol based on diffuse concave elevation without confirming the pericarditis pattern.
Non-diagnostic ECG with compelling story	Is the ECG normal or non-diagnostic, but the clinical presentation is convincingly ischemic?	Serial ECGs every 15-30 minutes (capture during symptoms). Serial troponins at 0, 3, 6 hours. Never discharge or deprioritize based on a normal initial ECG in a compelling clinical presentation. Up to 20% of confirmed MIs have a normal initial ECG.

PE pathway	Is the presentation consistent with pulmonary embolism (dyspnea, hypoxia, pleuritic pain, risk factors), and the ECG shows S1Q3T3, new RBBB, or sinus tachycardia without another explanation?	PE workup: Wells score, D-dimer if low probability, CTPA if intermediate/high. ECG is supportive, not diagnostic for PE. A normal ECG does not exclude PE.

12.4 The Five Absolute Contraindications

Five drug-rhythm interactions in this book produce immediate, potentially fatal consequences when violated. These are not clinical preferences or risk-benefit tradeoffs — they are patient safety requirements. Every nurse who manages cardiac monitoring patients must be able to state all five from memory and must be prepared to hold a medication order based on any one of them before the physician arrives at the bedside.

Contraindication	The Danger	What to Do Instead
Nitrates (and morphine) in RV infarction (V4R-positive inferior STEMI)	The RV is preload-dependent. Nitrates remove preload → cardiac output falls → immediate severe hypotension that can precipitate cardiovascular collapse.	IV fluid boluses (500 mL NS) for hypotension. Vasopressors (norepinephrine) if fluids insufficient. Proceed with STEMI protocol (PCI). Never give NTG without V4R in inferior STEMI.
Adenosine, verapamil, diltiazem, digoxin, IV beta-blockers in pre-excited AF	These agents block the AV node → all AF impulses routed exclusively through the accessory pathway at 300+ bpm → VF.	Procainamide IV (stable). Unsynchronized defibrillation 200 J (unstable). Recognize wide + irregular + > 200 bpm + WPW before any medication is given.

Amiodarone for torsades de pointes	Amiodarone further prolongs the QT interval. The drug that causes torsades cannot treat torsades.	IV $MgSO_4$ 2 g over 5-15 min (first-line regardless of serum Mg^{2+} level). Hold ALL QTc-prolonging medications. Overdrive pacing at 90-100 bpm if torsades recurs. Do not give amiodarone.
Cardioversion in digoxin toxicity	The toxic myocardium has a dramatically lowered VF threshold. Cardioversion energy can trigger immediate VF in a digoxin-toxic patient.	Hold digoxin immediately. Replete K^+ aggressively (target ≥4.0 mEq/L). Digibind (digoxin immune Fab) for hemodynamically significant toxicity. Defibrillation for confirmed VF (this is acceptable even in digoxin toxicity).
Stress testing in Wellens syndrome	The critical LAD stenosis has temporarily reperfused. Exercise-induced ischemia during a stress test can trigger re-occlusion and massive anterior STEMI in the treadmill room.	Cancel or hold the stress test order. Communicate the Wellens pattern to the physician by name. NPO status. Urgent cardiology consultation for coronary angiography. Document the stress test hold.

12.5 The Speed Drill — 15 ECG Clues, 5 Seconds Each

The following 15-item speed drill tests automaticity of recognition — the ability to identify the diagnosis and first action from the ECG clue alone, without working through the full 8-step method. This is the level of pattern recognition that experienced cardiac nurses reach after months of monitored practice. Cover the Diagnosis and Action columns, read the clue, state your answer aloud, then reveal. Target: 5 seconds per item.

#	ECG / Clinical Clue	Diagnosis	First Action
1	**Wide + irregular + > 220 bpm + WPW history**	Pre-excited AF	Procainamide IV (stable) / unsynchronized 200 J (unstable). Hold ALL AV nodal blockers.
2	**Deep symmetric T inversions V2-V3 in a pain-free patient**	Wellens syndrome (Type A)	Hold stress test. NPO. Urgent cardiology consult for angiography.
3	**Upsloping ST depression + tall peaked T waves V1-V4 with chest pain**	De Winter pattern	STEMI-equivalent activation. Cath lab now.
4	**Diffuse ST depression ≥6 leads + ST elevation in aVR only**	Left main / severe multivessel	Urgent angiography, same urgency as STEMI. Not 'serial troponins.'
5	**Inferior STEMI (II/III/aVF) + V4R: 1.8 mm ST elevation**	RV infarction	Hold nitrates. IV fluid boluses for hypotension. Proceed with PCI.
6	**Post-PCI wide regular rhythm at 72 bpm, LBBB morphology, appeared immediately after balloon inflation**	AIVR (reperfusion arrhythmia)	Do NOT treat. Document and observe. This is a benign reperfusion marker.

7	**Beat-to-beat QRS amplitude alternation + low voltage + JVD + muffled sounds + malignancy**	Cardiac tamponade	Bedside echo immediately. Prepare pericardiocentesis. Do not order troponin first.
8	**New coved ST elevation V1-V2 in a sedated patient on propofol > 48 hours**	Propofol infusion syndrome (PRIS)	Stop propofol immediately. Switch sedation. Check CK, lactate.
9	**Sine-wave QRS-T pattern + K^+ = 8.9 mEq/L + ESRD + missed dialysis**	Stage 4 hyperkalemia	IV calcium gluconate NOW. IV insulin + D50W. Emergency dialysis.
10	**New NPJT + regularized AF + digoxin level 3.1 + K^+ 2.8**	Digoxin toxicity	Hold digoxin. IV K^+ aggressively. Digibind. NEVER cardiovert.
11	**Diffuse concave ST elevation + PR depression in most leads + PR elevation in aVR + 3 weeks post-cardiac surgery**	Postpericardiotom y syndrome	NSAIDs + colchicine. Do NOT activate STEMI protocol.
12	**ST depression V1-V2 + tall R in V1 + no ST elevation anywhere + chest pain**	Posterior MI	Obtain V7-V9 immediately (≥0.5 mm = posterior STEMI-equivalent).

13	**Regular narrow-complex tachycardia at 220-300 bpm in a 4-month-old infant**	Pediatric SVT	Ice to face (dive reflex). If persists: adenosine 0.1 mg/kg rapid IV push.
14	**VT at 182 bpm, BP 74/40, patient confused and diaphoretic**	Unstable VT with pulse	Synchronized cardioversion 100 J, SYNC ON. Sedate if time allows.
15	**Complete AV block, wide ventricular escape at 28 bpm, BP 64/38**	Infranodal complete AV block	TCP immediately. Do NOT give atropine first. Atropine will not work.

12.6 The Shift-End Checklist

The shift-end checklist confirms that every cardiac monitoring responsibility has been fulfilled before the outgoing nurse transfers care. It is not a documentation form — it is a clinical habit that creates a safe handoff for every monitored cardiac patient on the unit.

SHIFT-END CARDIAC MONITORING CHECKLIST — COMPLETE FOR EVERY MONITORED PATIENT:

1. RHYTHM: Can you state the patient's current rhythm by name? Not 'looks fine' — the specific rhythm name, rate, and QRS width. If you cannot name it: obtain a 12-lead ECG before handing off.

2. EVENTS: Were there any significant rhythm events during your shift? Every event must be documented with time, description, intervention, response, and provider notification. No undocumented events should transfer to the next nurse.

3. CSTM: Is CSTM running for any patient who requires it? What is the current ST trend value in each monitored lead? Has there been any ST change from baseline during your shift, and is it addressed?

4. QTc: What is the current QTc for each patient on QTc-prolonging medications? Is it above 0.44 s? Above 0.50 s? Has any new QTc-prolonging drug been added this shift? Are the electrolyte targets (K^+ ≥4.0, Mg^{2+} ≥2.0) being met?

5. MEDICATIONS: Have any cardiac medications been started, stopped, changed, or held this shift? Is the receiving nurse explicitly aware of each change and its rationale? Are any orders pending clarification?
6. ALARMS: Are the alarm thresholds set appropriately for each patient's known baseline? Are any non-default thresholds in use, and does the receiving nurse understand why?
7. DEVICES: For pacemaker patients: are wire connections secure, are the settings documented, and is the most recent capture threshold check documented? For post-implant patients: are activity restrictions reinforced?
8. COMMUNICATIONS: Are all provider notifications documented with time, name, and response? Are there any outstanding follow-up items expected from cardiology or the covering physician during the next shift?

12.7 The Complete Bedside Read — One Page Reference

The following single-page reference integrates the 10-second triage, the 8-step method, the five branch points, and the five absolute contraindications into one visual sequence. This is the reference a nurse can return to at any point in their practice — whether reviewing after a difficult case, preparing for a new role, or teaching a student.

THE COMPLETE BEDSIDE READ — BOOK 5 INTEGRATED METHOD

PHASE 1 — 10-SECOND TRIAGE (before anything else)

• Pulseless? → CPR + ACLS immediately
• Life-threatening rhythm (VF, pulseless VT, asystole)? → Act now
• Immediate action needed (hemodynamically unstable brady/tachy, high-risk pattern visible)? → Act while getting 12-lead

PHASE 2 — 8-STEP SYSTEMATIC READ (~80 seconds)

1. Rate/rhythm → 2. Axis → 3. Intervals (QRS > 0.12 s? STOP → go to Step 5 first) → 4. Chamber enlargement → 5. QRS morphology / BBB (LBBB or paced? → Sgarbossa criteria for Steps 6-7) → 6. ST segment → 7. T waves → 8. Clinical correlation

PHASE 3 — FIVE BRANCH POINTS (run all five before declaring complete)

1. Standard STEMI criteria (no BBB): regional elevation + reciprocal → cath lab. Inferior → V4R before NTG.
2. Sgarbossa (LBBB/paced): concordant elevation ≥1 mm (Rule 1), concordant depression ≥1 mm V1-V3 (Rule 2), or ratio ≤ −0.25 (Rule 3 modified) → STEMI-equivalent.
3. Pericarditis: diffuse concave elevation + PR depression + NO reciprocal changes → NSAIDs + colchicine, not cath lab.
4. Non-diagnostic ECG + compelling story → serial ECGs during symptoms + serial troponins. Never discharge.
5. PE pathway: dyspnea + hypoxia + S1Q3T3/new RBBB/sinus tachycardia → Wells → D-dimer or CTPA.

PHASE 4 — FIVE ABSOLUTE CONTRAINDICATIONS (check before every medication)

1. Nitrates in V4R-positive RV infarction → IV fluids instead.
2. Adenosine / verapamil / diltiazem / digoxin / IV beta-blockers in pre-excited AF → procainamide or defibrillation.
3. Amiodarone for torsades → IV $MgSO_4$ 2 g instead.
4. Cardioversion in digoxin toxicity → Digibind + K^+ repletion instead.
5. Stress test in Wellens syndrome → cancel the test, urgent angiography instead.

PHASE 5 — COMMUNICATE (every significant finding)

SBAR: name the rhythm + rate + QRS width + BP + stability in the first sentence. Read back every verbal order. Document time of finding, provider name, time of notification, response, intervention, and patient response.

PHASE 6 — DOCUMENT AND HAND OFF

Real-time documentation: finding → assessment → action → notification → response. Shift-end checklist: rhythm named, events documented, CSTM current, QTc checked, medications reconciled, alarms individualized, devices confirmed, communications documented.

12.8 Final Note — What This Book Has Built

Every chapter in this book addressed a different setting, a different patient population, or a different category of ECG finding. But the underlying clinical skill being built in every chapter was the same: the ability to look at a cardiac monitor, apply a consistent sequence, and take the right action — without hesitation, without omitting a safety step, and without needing to find a reference.

That skill is not primarily a knowledge skill. It is a sequence skill. The nurse who has run the 10-second triage, the 8-step read, the five branch points, and the contraindication check on enough patients will eventually do it automatically — in the same way that an experienced driver checks mirrors, blind spots, and speed without consciously thinking about the sequence. The sequence becomes the reflex.

Book 5 built that sequence for the highest-acuity cardiac monitoring environments in clinical practice. The emergency department patient with crushing chest pain. The ICU patient with a sine-wave QRS at 3 AM. The post-cardiac surgery patient with a new rhythm on post-operative day 2. The ward patient whose Mobitz II appears on telemetry at shift change. The pregnant patient in cardiac arrest. Each of these scenarios has a specific, teachable, repeatable correct response. This book has provided that response for each of them.

The shift-end checklist is the last clinical act in this book. It is also the most important daily habit it recommends. The nurse who completes it faithfully — naming every rhythm, documenting every event, checking every QTc, reconciling every cardiac medication, and confirming every device — is practicing at the standard that prevents the adverse events that harm patients in monitored settings. That standard is the goal of the ECG in 60 Minutes series from Book 1 through Book 6.

> **BEDSIDE PEARL** The method is the discipline. Not the knowledge of what VT looks like, or what Wellens syndrome means, or when to apply Sgarbossa criteria — those are facts that this series has provided across five books. The discipline is running the same sequence every time, on every ECG, whether the patient is a straightforward sinus rhythm check or the most complex post-cardiac surgery case on the unit. The sequence protects patients because it runs even when cognitive load is high, the unit is busy, and the easy path is to glance at the monitor and assume it looks fine. Run the sequence. Name the rhythm. Check the branch points. Verify the contraindications. Communicate the finding. Document the response. That is the complete bedside read from monitor to action.

KEY POINTS — CHAPTER 12

The Integrated Method

- Six phases in order: 10-second triage → 8-step systematic read → five branch points → five contraindication checks → SBAR communication → documentation and handoff. The sequence does not vary based on setting or apparent urgency.
- Step 5 (BBB check) must precede Step 6 (ST reading). LBBB or paced rhythm → Sgarbossa criteria replace standard STEMI thresholds. This single sequence point prevents the most dangerous misdiagnoses in acute cardiology.

Five Branch Points

- Run all five before declaring any ECG complete: standard STEMI, Sgarbossa, pericarditis differential, non-diagnostic ECG + compelling story, PE pathway. One missed branch point is one missed diagnosis.

Five Contraindications

- Nitrates in V4R-positive RV infarction. AV nodal blockers in pre-excited AF. Amiodarone for torsades. Cardioversion in digoxin toxicity. Stress test in Wellens syndrome. Memorize all five. Hold the medication order before the physician arrives if any one applies.

Speed Drill and Shift-End Checklist

- Speed drill: 15 items, 5 seconds each. If any item takes more than 10 seconds, that pattern requires additional focused practice.
- Shift-end checklist: rhythm named, events documented, CSTM current, QTc checked, medications reconciled, alarms individualized, devices confirmed, communications documented. Every monitored patient, every shift.

REMEMBER THIS

✓ The sequence is the safety net. A nurse who runs the same 6-phase method on every ECG — even the routine ones — will run it correctly when the difficult case arrives. A nurse who takes shortcuts on the routine cases will take the same shortcuts on the case where the shortcut causes harm. The 10-second triage, the 8-step read, the five branch points, and the contraindication check together take less than 3 minutes on a straightforward ECG. The investment is 3 minutes to ensure nothing is missed. That investment compounds across every shift into a standard of care that protects patients.

✓ The five absolute contraindications are patient safety interventions, not clinical preferences. When a medication order is given that violates one of the five, the nurse's professional obligation is to hold the order, communicate the contraindication to the provider with a specific clinical rationale, and document the hold. This is the definition of nursing advocacy in the cardiac monitoring context. The nurse who holds the diltiazem in a pre-excited AF patient because she recognized the pattern before the physician arrived may have prevented a VF. That action will never appear in a case report, because the adverse event did not occur.

✓ The shift-end checklist is the last safety check before care is transferred. The 60 minutes after shift change is the highest-risk window for monitored cardiac patients. A receiving nurse who is fully informed from the first minute of the shift — with every rhythm named, every event documented, every QTc value known, every cardiac medication change communicated — is a receiving nurse who can respond correctly if something happens in the first hour. The checklist creates that nurse at the start of every shift.

www.ingramcontent.com/pod-product-compliance
Lightning Source LLC
LaVergne TN
LVHW010726061126
851857LV00014B/1361
* 9 7 9 2 4 0 6 7 6 2 2 8 6 *